Materials for Tissue Engineering: Building a Better Tomorrow

Shane Hector

Copyright © [2023]

Title: Materials for Tissue Engineering: Building a Better Tomorrow

Author's: Shane Hector

All rights reserved. No part of this publication may be reproduced, stored in a retrieval system, or transmitted in any form or by any means, electronic, mechanical, photocopying, recording, or otherwise, without the prior written permission of the publisher or author, except in the case of brief quotations embodied in critical reviews and certain other non-commercial uses permitted by copyright law.

This book was printed and published by [Publisher's: **Shane Hector**] in [2023]

ISBN:

TABLE OF CONTENT

Chapter 1: Introduction to Tissue Engineering   09

Definition and Overview of Tissue Engineering

Historical Background

Importance and Potential of Tissue Engineering

Challenges and Limitations in Tissue Engineering

Chapter 2: Fundamentals of Biomedical Materials   17

Introduction to Biomedical Materials

Classification of Biomedical Materials

Properties and Requirements of Biomedical Materials

Biocompatibility and Biodegradability

Chapter 3: Biomaterials for Tissue Engineering   25

Introduction to Biomaterials

Natural Biomaterials

Collagen

Gelatin

Chitosan

Synthetic Biomaterials

Polymers

Ceramics

Metals

Composites

Biomimetic and Bioactive Materials

Surface Modification Techniques

Scaffolds and Tissue Matrices

Chapter 4: Materials for Medical Devices and Implants   52

Introduction to Medical Devices and Implants

Metallic Materials for Medical Devices

Stainless Steel

Titanium Alloys

Cobalt-Chromium Alloys

Polymeric Materials for Medical Devices

Polyethylene

Silicone

Polyurethane

Ceramic Materials for Medical Devices

Alumina

Zirconia

Hydroxyapatite

Chapter 5: Engineering Approaches in Tissue Engineering 78

Scaffold Fabrication Techniques

Salt Leaching

Electrospinning

3D Printing

Cell Seeding and Culturing Techniques

Static Seeding

Perfusion Bioreactors

Co-culture Techniques

Tissue Engineering Strategies

In vitro Engineering

In vivo Engineering

Ex vivo Engineering

Chapter 6: Applications of Tissue Engineering 104

Skin Tissue Engineering

Burns and Wound Healing

Skin Grafts

Artificial Skin Substitutes

Bone Tissue Engineering

Bone Defect Repair

Bone Grafts and Substitutes

Osteochondral Tissue Engineering

Cartilage Tissue Engineering

Articular Cartilage Repair

Meniscus Repair

Organ and Vascular Tissue Engineering

Liver Tissue Engineering

Heart Tissue Engineering

Blood Vessel Engineering

Chapter 7: Regulatory and Ethical Considerations in Tissue Engineering   135

Regulatory Frameworks and Approval Process

Ethical Considerations in Tissue Engineering Research

Future Challenges and Directions in Tissue Engineering

Chapter 8: Conclusion and Future Outlook   141

Summary of Key Findings

Promising Developments and Emerging Trends

Impact of Tissue Engineering on Healthcare

The Role of Materials in Shaping a Better Tomorrow

Chapter 1: Introduction to Tissue Engineering

Definition and Overview of Tissue Engineering

Tissue engineering is an interdisciplinary field that combines principles from materials science, engineering, biology, and medicine to develop artificial tissues and organs for transplantation. It involves the application of engineering principles to design, create, and manipulate biological materials that can replace or restore the function of damaged or diseased tissues in the human body.

The field of tissue engineering emerged in the late 1980s, and since then, it has revolutionized the way we think about regenerative medicine and the possibilities for treating various medical conditions. By understanding the principles of tissue engineering, researchers and scientists have been able to create functional tissues, such as skin, cartilage, bone, and even complex organs like the liver and heart.

The main goal of tissue engineering is to develop functional tissues that can integrate seamlessly with the recipient's body, providing long-term solutions for patients suffering from organ failure, tissue damage, or congenital abnormalities. This innovative approach aims to overcome the limitations of traditional transplantation methods, including organ shortages, rejection issues, and the need for lifelong immunosuppression.

Materials science and engineering play a crucial role in tissue engineering. By designing and fabricating biomaterials, researchers can create scaffolds that mimic the structure and function of native tissues. These scaffolds serve as a framework for cells to grow and differentiate into functional tissues. They can be made from a wide range of materials, including polymers, ceramics, metals, and composites, each with their unique properties and advantages.

In addition to scaffolds, tissue engineering also involves the use of bioactive molecules, such as growth factors and cytokines, to stimulate cell growth and promote tissue regeneration. These molecules can be incorporated into the scaffolds or delivered through controlled release systems to enhance the healing process.

Tissue engineering has the potential to revolutionize healthcare by providing personalized solutions for patients in need of tissue or organ replacement. It offers the possibility of customizing therapies based on individual patient needs, reducing the risks associated with transplantation and improving overall patient outcomes.

In conclusion, tissue engineering is an exciting and rapidly advancing field that holds great promise for the future of regenerative medicine. By combining principles from materials science and engineering with biological knowledge, researchers are working towards building a better tomorrow, where functional tissues and organs can be engineered to improve the quality of life for millions of people worldwide.

Historical Background

In order to appreciate the advancements made in tissue engineering today, it is crucial to understand the historical background that shaped this field. Tissue engineering, as we know it today, is the result of centuries of scientific discoveries and innovative breakthroughs in the field of materials science and engineering.

The roots of tissue engineering can be traced back to ancient civilizations such as the Egyptians and Greeks, who experimented with natural materials to heal wounds and restore damaged tissues. However, it was not until the 19th century that significant progress was made in the development of materials and techniques for tissue regeneration.

One of the key milestones in tissue engineering was the discovery of biocompatible materials. In the early 1900s, scientists began exploring the use of materials such as ceramics, metals, and polymers to replace or repair damaged tissues. These materials were designed to mimic the properties of natural tissues and provide a supportive framework for cell growth and regeneration.

The breakthroughs in biomaterials during the mid-20th century paved the way for the development of artificial organs and prosthetics. Scientists realized that by combining the right materials with living cells, they could create functional tissues and organs. This led to the birth of tissue engineering as a distinct field of research in the 1980s.

Since then, tissue engineering has witnessed a rapid evolution, thanks to advancements in materials science and engineering. Researchers have been able to design and fabricate scaffolds with precise structural and mechanical properties, allowing cells to attach, proliferate, and differentiate into functional tissues.

In recent years, the field of tissue engineering has expanded beyond the repair and replacement of tissues. Scientists are now exploring the potential of engineered tissues in drug testing, disease modeling, and regenerative medicine. The development of bioactive materials, such as hydrogels and nanomaterials, has further enhanced the capabilities of tissue engineering, enabling the controlled release of growth factors and therapeutic agents.

As we delve into the fascinating world of tissue engineering, it is important to acknowledge the contributions of materials science and engineering in shaping this field. The historical background provides a context for understanding the challenges and opportunities that lie ahead in building a better tomorrow for tissue engineering. By harnessing the power of materials, scientists are unlocking new possibilities in regenerative medicine and paving the way for innovative solutions to complex medical problems.

In conclusion, the historical background of tissue engineering highlights the transformative journey that this field has undergone, from ancient civilizations to modern-day advancements. As we continue to push the boundaries of materials science and engineering, the future of tissue engineering holds immense promise for improving healthcare and enhancing the lives of individuals worldwide.

Importance and Potential of Tissue Engineering

Tissue engineering represents a revolutionary field that combines principles from materials science and engineering to address critical challenges in healthcare. This subchapter will explore the importance and potential of tissue engineering, discussing its impact on both patients and the field of materials science and engineering.

At its core, tissue engineering aims to develop functional replacement tissues and organs, providing hope for countless patients suffering from organ failure, tissue damage, or congenital defects. The ability to regenerate damaged or lost tissues would significantly improve the quality of life for individuals and reduce the burden on healthcare systems worldwide. Tissue engineering offers the promise of personalized medicine, as it allows for the creation of patient-specific tissues, reducing the risk of immune rejection and enhancing the success rate of transplants.

Materials science and engineering play a crucial role in tissue engineering by providing suitable biomaterials that support cell growth and tissue regeneration. These biomaterials act as scaffolds, mimicking the natural extracellular matrix and providing mechanical support to cells. By selecting and designing materials with specific properties, such as biocompatibility, biodegradability, and mechanical strength, researchers can create optimal environments for tissue growth and regeneration.

Moreover, materials scientists are continuously exploring innovative strategies to enhance the functional properties of engineered tissues. Researchers are incorporating bioactive molecules, such as growth factors and cytokines, into biomaterials to promote cell adhesion, proliferation, and differentiation. Additionally, the integration of nanotechnology and advanced manufacturing techniques allows for the development of intricate tissue architectures, enabling the recreation of complex tissues like blood vessels or even organs.

The potential of tissue engineering extends beyond regenerative medicine. By providing in vitro models that closely mimic human tissues, tissue engineering is revolutionizing drug discovery and toxicology testing. These models allow for more accurate and ethical testing, reducing the reliance on animal models and improving the safety and efficacy of pharmaceuticals.

In conclusion, tissue engineering is a rapidly evolving field that holds immense importance and potential for both patients and the materials science and engineering community. By leveraging materials science principles, tissue engineering offers hope for patients in need of tissue and organ replacements. Furthermore, it contributes to the advancement of materials science and engineering by pushing the boundaries of biomaterial design and fabrication techniques. As we continue to unravel the complexities of tissue engineering, we move closer to building a better tomorrow for patients worldwide.

Challenges and Limitations in Tissue Engineering

In the field of tissue engineering, remarkable advancements have been made in recent years, offering hope for a better tomorrow in regenerative medicine. However, it is essential to acknowledge that there are still challenges and limitations that need to be overcome. This subchapter aims to shed light on these obstacles and provide insights into the future directions of tissue engineering.

1. Biomaterial Selection: Selecting the appropriate biomaterials for tissue engineering is crucial. The material must possess suitable mechanical properties, biocompatibility, and degradation characteristics. Additionally, it should promote cell adhesion, proliferation, and differentiation. Achieving this delicate balance remains a challenge.

2. Vascularization: The successful integration of engineered tissues with the host's blood vessels is essential for their survival and functionality. However, creating a complex vascular network within the engineered tissue remains challenging. Ensuring a sufficient blood supply to support cell growth, nutrient exchange, and waste removal is a major hurdle.

3. Immune Response: The immune system plays a crucial role in tissue rejection. Although biocompatible materials are used, the immune response can still lead to tissue rejection or failure. Developing strategies to modulate the immune response and promote tissue acceptance is a significant challenge.

4. Tissue Complexity: Different tissues in the human body possess unique characteristics, making their regeneration a complex task. For

example, engineering the intricate structure of the heart or the complexity of the brain presents substantial challenges. Overcoming these limitations requires advancements in biomaterial design, cell sourcing, and tissue fabrication techniques.

5. Scale-up and Manufacturing: While tissue engineering has shown success on a small scale, translating these achievements to large-scale production remains a challenge. The development of scalable manufacturing processes is crucial for the widespread application of tissue-engineered constructs.

6. Regulatory Hurdles: The translation of tissue engineering from the laboratory to clinical practice is subject to rigorous regulatory frameworks. Meeting the safety and efficacy standards set by regulatory authorities is a significant limitation. Streamlining these processes and ensuring faster approval of tissue-engineered constructs is necessary for their timely implementation.

Looking ahead, interdisciplinary collaborations, advancements in biomaterial science, and novel fabrication techniques hold promise in addressing these challenges. Researchers in the field of materials science and engineering play a vital role in developing innovative biomaterials and manufacturing processes to overcome the limitations of tissue engineering.

By understanding and addressing these challenges, we can pave the way for a future where tissue engineering revolutionizes healthcare, offering regenerative solutions for patients worldwide. Together, we can build a better tomorrow, where tissue engineering plays a pivotal role in restoring and improving human health.

Chapter 2: Fundamentals of Biomedical Materials

Introduction to Biomedical Materials

In the field of tissue engineering, the development and use of biomedical materials play a vital role in advancing healthcare solutions. These materials are specifically designed to interact with biological systems, aiming to repair or replace damaged tissues and organs. This subchapter provides an introduction to the fascinating world of biomedical materials, exploring their importance, types, and applications.

Biomedical materials are engineered substances that are biocompatible, meaning they can integrate seamlessly with living tissues without causing adverse reactions. They are carefully designed to possess specific physical and chemical properties that mimic the natural environment of the body. These materials can be classified into three major categories: metals and alloys, polymers, and ceramics.

Metals and alloys are widely used in medical devices, such as orthopedic implants and dental fixtures, due to their excellent mechanical properties and corrosion resistance. Titanium and stainless steel are common examples of metals used in these applications. Polymers, on the other hand, are versatile materials that can be tailored to mimic the properties of natural tissues. They are commonly used in scaffolds for tissue engineering, drug delivery systems, and wound dressings. Examples of biomedical polymers include poly(lactic-co-glycolic acid) (PLGA) and polyethylene glycol (PEG).

Ceramics, such as hydroxyapatite and bioglass, are biocompatible materials that are commonly used in bone tissue engineering. They possess excellent bioactivity and can promote bone regeneration when implanted in the body. In addition to these three major categories, composite materials, which combine different materials, are also extensively used in biomedical applications. These composites can provide enhanced mechanical properties, improved biocompatibility, and controlled drug release.

The field of tissue engineering aims to create functional tissues and organs by combining cells, scaffolds, and signaling factors. Biomedical materials serve as the scaffolds upon which cells can grow and differentiate into the desired tissue type. These materials provide mechanical support, guide cell behavior, and allow for the exchange of nutrients and waste products. They must possess suitable porosity, surface chemistry, and mechanical properties to support cell attachment, proliferation, and tissue regeneration.

In conclusion, biomedical materials are crucial components in the field of tissue engineering and have revolutionized the medical industry. They offer the potential for regenerative medicine, personalized healthcare, and improved quality of life for patients. This subchapter provides a comprehensive overview of the different types of biomedical materials and their applications in the field of tissue engineering, making it a valuable resource for individuals interested in the field of materials science and engineering.

Classification of Biomedical Materials

In the field of tissue engineering, the development and utilization of various materials play a crucial role in achieving successful outcomes. Materials used in this field are designed to interact with biological systems, promoting tissue regeneration and ultimately improving the quality of life for patients. Understanding the classification of biomedical materials is vital for researchers, scientists, and engineers working in the field of tissue engineering.

Biomedical materials are classified based on their composition, structure, and function. This classification allows researchers to categorize materials and select the most suitable ones for specific applications. Here, we will explore the different categories of biomedical materials and their significance in tissue engineering.

The first category is natural materials, which are derived from biological sources such as collagen, chitosan, and silk. These materials possess excellent biocompatibility and bioactivity, making them ideal for tissue engineering applications. Natural materials can mimic the extracellular matrix, providing a favorable environment for cell attachment, proliferation, and differentiation.

The second category is synthetic materials, which are chemically engineered to possess specific properties. Examples include polymers like poly(lactic acid) (PLA), poly(glycolic acid) (PGA), and their copolymer poly(lactic-co-glycolic acid) (PLGA). Synthetic materials offer controllable mechanical properties, degradation rates, and surface characteristics, allowing researchers to tailor them according to the requirements of a specific tissue.

The third category is composite materials, which combine natural and synthetic materials to leverage their individual advantages. These materials can harness the bioactivity of natural materials and the mechanical integrity of synthetic materials. For example, a composite scaffold may consist of a natural material like collagen and a synthetic material like PLA, providing both biocompatibility and structural support.

Another category is metallic materials, such as titanium and its alloys, stainless steel, and cobalt-chromium alloys. These materials possess excellent mechanical strength and corrosion resistance, making them suitable for load-bearing applications, such as orthopedic implants.

Lastly, there are ceramic materials, which include hydroxyapatite and tricalcium phosphate. These materials closely resemble the mineral composition of human bone and are commonly used in bone tissue engineering. Ceramic materials can provide a scaffold for new bone growth and facilitate the integration of implants with natural tissue.

Understanding the classification of biomedical materials allows researchers to select the most appropriate materials for their specific tissue engineering applications. By carefully choosing materials, scientists can enhance the success rate of tissue regeneration and ultimately improve the lives of patients. The ongoing research and development in this field hold great promise for building a better tomorrow in the field of tissue engineering.

Properties and Requirements of Biomedical Materials

Biomedical materials play a crucial role in the field of tissue engineering, where the goal is to create functional and biocompatible replacements for damaged or diseased tissues and organs. These materials are designed to support the growth and regeneration of cells, while also possessing specific properties that allow them to integrate seamlessly with the natural tissues in the body. In this subchapter, we will explore the properties and requirements of biomedical materials, highlighting their importance in the field of tissue engineering.

One of the key properties of biomedical materials is biocompatibility. This refers to the ability of a material to perform its intended function without eliciting any adverse reactions or toxic effects within the body. Biocompatible materials are non-toxic, non-allergenic, and do not induce an immune response. They should also be able to degrade over time, as the regenerated tissue gradually takes over its function.

Another important property is mechanical strength. Biomedical materials should have sufficient strength to withstand the physiological forces exerted on them, ensuring their stability and longevity within the body. The mechanical properties of these materials can be tailored to match those of the surrounding tissues, allowing for seamless integration.

Furthermore, the surface characteristics of biomedical materials are crucial for cellular adhesion and proliferation. The materials should possess appropriate surface roughness, porosity, and chemistry to facilitate cell attachment, migration, and growth. Surface modifications, such as the addition of bioactive molecules or coatings, can further enhance these interactions.

In addition to biocompatibility and mechanical strength, biomedical materials must also be bioresorbable to a certain extent. Depending on the application, the material should degrade over time, allowing the regenerated tissue to take over its function. This property is particularly important in temporary scaffolds, which provide a framework for tissue growth and eventually degrade as the tissue regenerates.

To meet the requirements of tissue engineering applications, biomedical materials can be made from various sources. Natural materials, such as collagen, chitosan, and hyaluronic acid, offer excellent biocompatibility but may have limited mechanical properties. Synthetic materials, such as polyesters and hydrogels, can be precisely engineered to have specific characteristics, including mechanical strength and degradation rate. Hybrid materials, combining natural and synthetic components, can offer a balance between biocompatibility and mechanical properties.

In conclusion, the properties and requirements of biomedical materials are critical factors in the success of tissue engineering. Biocompatibility, mechanical strength, surface characteristics, and bioresorbability are some of the key considerations when developing these materials. By understanding and optimizing these properties, researchers and engineers can build a better tomorrow by creating materials that promote the regeneration and restoration of damaged or diseased tissues.

Biocompatibility and Biodegradability

In the field of tissue engineering, the successful development of biomaterials that are both biocompatible and biodegradable is crucial for building a better tomorrow. These materials play a significant role in the creation of functional tissue substitutes, organ regeneration, and medical devices. This subchapter explores the concepts of biocompatibility and biodegradability, highlighting their importance and providing an overview of the advancements in materials science and engineering.

Biocompatibility refers to the ability of a material to perform its intended function within a specific application without causing any adverse reactions or harm to the biological system. When designing materials for tissue engineering, it is essential to choose substances that are compatible with the host organism, ensuring minimal immune response and promoting cell adhesion, proliferation, and differentiation. Various factors, such as surface properties, mechanical strength, and degradation characteristics, influence the biocompatibility of a material.

On the other hand, biodegradability refers to the ability of a material to break down over time into harmless byproducts that can be metabolized or excreted by the body. This property is particularly important in tissue engineering, as it allows the scaffolds or implants to gradually degrade and be replaced by newly formed tissue. Biodegradable materials can eliminate the need for surgical removal procedures and enable the regeneration of functional tissue.

Materials science and engineering have made significant strides in developing biocompatible and biodegradable materials for tissue engineering applications. Synthetic polymers such as poly(lactic-co-glycolic acid) (PLGA), poly(ethylene glycol) (PEG), and polycaprolactone (PCL) have gained immense popularity due to their tunable properties, degradation kinetics, and ability to support cell growth. Natural materials, including collagen, chitosan, and alginate, have also been extensively investigated for their biocompatibility and ability to mimic the extracellular matrix.

Researchers have explored various techniques to enhance the biocompatibility and biodegradability of these materials. Surface modifications, such as coating with bioactive molecules or creating nanotopographies, can improve cell-material interactions and promote tissue regeneration. Additionally, incorporating bioactive agents, growth factors, or drugs into the material matrix can further enhance the therapeutic potential of these biomaterials.

In conclusion, biocompatibility and biodegradability are critical considerations in the development of materials for tissue engineering. Advancements in materials science and engineering have led to the creation of biocompatible and biodegradable materials that can support cell growth and tissue regeneration. These materials hold immense promise for the field of tissue engineering, offering the potential to build a better tomorrow by providing functional tissue substitutes and enabling organ regeneration. By further exploring and refining these properties, scientists and engineers can continue to revolutionize the field and improve patient outcomes.

Chapter 3: Biomaterials for Tissue Engineering

Introduction to Biomaterials

Biomaterials play a crucial role in the field of tissue engineering, revolutionizing the way we approach medical treatments and healthcare. This subchapter will provide a comprehensive introduction to biomaterials, covering their definition, types, properties, and applications. Whether you are a student, researcher, medical professional, or simply curious about materials science and engineering, this content aims to provide a solid foundation in understanding biomaterials and their significance in building a better tomorrow.

Biomaterials can be defined as any substance, natural or synthetic, that is engineered to interact with biological systems for medical purposes. They are designed to mimic the properties of living tissues and organs, promoting tissue regeneration and restoring normal physiological functions. With advancements in materials science and engineering, researchers have developed a wide range of biomaterials with unique characteristics suitable for various medical applications.

This subchapter will explore the different types of biomaterials, including metals, ceramics, polymers, and composites. Each material has its own set of advantages and limitations, making it suitable for specific applications. For instance, metals such as titanium are widely used in orthopedic implants due to their strength and biocompatibility. On the other hand, polymers like poly(lactic-co-glycolic acid) (PLGA) are commonly used in drug delivery systems due to their biodegradability and tunable properties.

Understanding the properties of biomaterials is crucial for their successful integration into the human body. This subchapter will delve into the mechanical, chemical, and biological properties of biomaterials, discussing how these properties can be tailored to meet specific requirements. Additionally, it will cover the concept of biocompatibility, ensuring that biomaterials do not elicit adverse reactions from the body and are safe for long-term use.

Lastly, this subchapter will shed light on the diverse applications of biomaterials in tissue engineering. From regenerating damaged tissues to creating artificial organs and scaffolds, biomaterials have paved the way for groundbreaking medical advancements. Examples of successful applications, such as bone grafts, skin substitutes, and cardiovascular stents, will be discussed, highlighting the impact of biomaterials on improving patient outcomes and quality of life.

In conclusion, this subchapter serves as a comprehensive introduction to biomaterials, covering their definition, types, properties, and applications. It is aimed at a diverse audience, including students, researchers, medical professionals, and anyone interested in materials science and engineering. By understanding the fundamentals of biomaterials, we can unlock their potential to build a better tomorrow in the field of tissue engineering and healthcare.

Natural Biomaterials

In the field of tissue engineering, the search for suitable materials that can mimic and support the functions of native tissues has been a constant endeavor. One promising avenue of research is the exploration of natural biomaterials, which are derived from plants, animals, and other natural sources. These materials offer unique advantages in terms of biocompatibility, bioactivity, and mechanical properties, making them highly attractive for tissue engineering applications.

One important class of natural biomaterials is extracellular matrix (ECM) components. ECM is the intricate network of proteins and carbohydrates that provides structural support and biochemical cues to cells in native tissues. By isolating and modifying ECM components, researchers can create scaffolds that closely resemble the natural environment of cells. These scaffolds can then be used to guide cell behavior and promote tissue regeneration. Examples of ECM-based biomaterials include collagen, elastin, and hyaluronic acid.

Collagen, the most abundant protein in the human body, has been extensively investigated for tissue engineering purposes. It possesses excellent biocompatibility and can be easily processed into various forms, such as gels, films, and fibers. Collagen scaffolds have shown great potential in the regeneration of skin, bone, cartilage, and blood vessels. Elastin, on the other hand, is a protein responsible for the elasticity of tissues such as the lungs and blood vessels. Elastin-based biomaterials have been developed to engineer tissues that require high stretchability, such as cardiac muscle and blood vessel walls.

Apart from proteins, polysaccharides also play a crucial role in natural biomaterials. Hyaluronic acid (HA), a glycosaminoglycan found in the ECM, has attracted significant attention in tissue engineering due to its biocompatibility, viscoelasticity, and ability to retain water. HA-based hydrogels have been utilized for wound healing, cartilage repair, and drug delivery. Chitosan, derived from the shells of crustaceans, is another polysaccharide with excellent biocompatibility and antimicrobial properties. Chitosan-based scaffolds have been explored for applications in bone, cartilage, and nerve tissue engineering.

The use of natural biomaterials in tissue engineering offers several advantages over synthetic materials. Natural biomaterials are often better tolerated by the body, reducing the risk of adverse reactions. They can also provide biochemical cues that promote cell adhesion, migration, and differentiation. Furthermore, natural biomaterials are biodegradable, allowing for the gradual regeneration of native tissues without the need for surgical removal.

In conclusion, natural biomaterials hold great promise for tissue engineering applications. Their ability to closely mimic the properties of native tissues, combined with their biocompatibility and bioactivity, make them ideal candidates for the development of advanced scaffolds. Continued research and innovation in the field of natural biomaterials will undoubtedly contribute to building a better tomorrow in tissue engineering, bringing us closer to the goal of restoring damaged or diseased tissues and improving the quality of life for countless individuals.

Collagen

Collagen: The Building Block of Tissue Engineering

Collagen is a fundamental component of tissue engineering, playing a vital role in the regeneration and repair of various tissues in the human body. This subchapter delves into the significance of collagen in materials science and engineering, exploring its properties, applications, and potential for building a better tomorrow.

Collagen, a versatile and abundant protein, is found in connective tissues such as tendons, ligaments, cartilage, and skin. Its unique structure and composition make it an excellent biomaterial for tissue engineering. The triple-helix structure of collagen provides strength and stability, while its high biocompatibility allows for integration with host tissues. Collagen also possesses bioactive properties that facilitate cell adhesion, migration, and differentiation, making it an ideal substrate for tissue regeneration.

In materials science and engineering, collagen can be derived from various sources, including animal tissues and recombinant technology. Its mechanical properties can be modified by crosslinking techniques, enabling the development of scaffolds with specific characteristics tailored to different tissue engineering applications. Collagen-based scaffolds provide a three-dimensional framework that supports cell growth, proliferation, and tissue formation. These scaffolds can be fabricated into various shapes and sizes, making them adaptable to different tissue regeneration needs.

One of the most promising applications of collagen in tissue engineering is in the field of wound healing. Collagen dressings promote the formation of new blood vessels, accelerate tissue regeneration, and enhance wound closure. In addition, collagen-based materials are being explored for the repair and regeneration of bone, cartilage, and cardiovascular tissues. The ability of collagen scaffolds to mimic the extracellular matrix and provide a suitable environment for cell attachment and proliferation makes them essential tools in tissue engineering.

However, despite its immense potential, there are challenges associated with the use of collagen in tissue engineering. Issues such as immunogenicity, biodegradation rate control, and mechanical stability need to be addressed to optimize collagen-based materials for clinical applications. Researchers and engineers in the field of materials science are actively working on improving collagen-based biomaterials to overcome these challenges and enhance their performance in tissue engineering.

In conclusion, collagen is a critical component of tissue engineering, offering immense potential for building a better tomorrow. Its unique properties, biocompatibility, and bioactive characteristics make it a versatile biomaterial for tissue regeneration and repair. Through continuous research and technological advancements, collagen-based materials can be optimized to revolutionize the field of tissue engineering, paving the way for improved healthcare and a brighter future for all.

Gelatin

Gelatin is a versatile and widely used material in the field of tissue engineering. Derived from collagen, a protein found in animal connective tissues, gelatin offers several unique properties that make it an ideal choice for various applications in this field.

One of the key advantages of gelatin is its biocompatibility. This means that it is well-tolerated by the human body and does not cause any adverse reactions when used in tissue engineering. Gelatin can be easily processed into different forms, such as hydrogels or scaffolds, which can mimic the natural environment of cells and support their growth and development.

The mechanical properties of gelatin can be tailored to suit specific tissue engineering needs. By adjusting the concentration or crosslinking of gelatin, the stiffness and elasticity of the material can be modified. This is crucial for mimicking the mechanical properties of different tissues in the body, such as soft tissues like skin or tough tissues like cartilage or bone.

Gelatin also possesses excellent cell adhesion properties, allowing cells to attach and spread on its surface. This is essential for promoting cell growth and tissue regeneration. Moreover, gelatin can be easily functionalized with bioactive molecules, such as growth factors or peptides, which can further enhance cell attachment and tissue formation.

In addition to its biocompatibility and mechanical properties, gelatin is also biodegradable. This means that it can be gradually broken down and absorbed by the body over time, as new tissue forms. This property eliminates the need for a second surgery to remove the material, making gelatin an attractive choice for tissue engineering applications.

Gelatin-based materials have been successfully used in a wide range of tissue engineering applications, including wound healing, bone regeneration, and cartilage repair. Ongoing research is also exploring its potential in developing bioartificial organs and tissues.

In conclusion, gelatin is a versatile and promising material for tissue engineering. Its biocompatibility, tunable mechanical properties, excellent cell adhesion, and biodegradability make it an ideal choice for creating scaffolds and hydrogels that can support and promote tissue regeneration. As the field of tissue engineering continues to advance, gelatin-based materials will play a crucial role in building a better tomorrow for regenerative medicine.

Chitosan

Chitosan: A Versatile Biomaterial for Tissue Engineering

Introduction:
Chitosan, a biocompatible and biodegradable biomaterial derived from chitin, has gained significant interest in the field of tissue engineering due to its unique properties and potential applications. This subchapter aims to provide a comprehensive overview of chitosan, highlighting its properties, fabrication methods, and various tissue engineering applications.

Properties and Fabrication Methods:
Chitosan possesses several advantageous properties that make it an attractive material for tissue engineering. These include biocompatibility, biodegradability, antimicrobial activity, and the ability to promote cell adhesion and proliferation. Chitosan can be fabricated into various forms, such as films, scaffolds, hydrogels, nanoparticles, and fibers, through different techniques including solvent casting, freeze-drying, electrospinning, and cross-linking.

Tissue Engineering Applications:
Chitosan-based biomaterials have found applications in a wide range of tissue engineering fields. In bone tissue engineering, chitosan scaffolds have been extensively studied for their ability to support osteogenesis and bone regeneration. Chitosan-based hydrogels have shown promise in cartilage tissue engineering, providing a suitable environment for chondrocyte growth and extracellular matrix synthesis. Additionally, chitosan nanoparticles have been explored for

drug delivery systems, enabling targeted and controlled release of therapeutic agents.

Challenges and Future Perspectives:
Despite the numerous advantages offered by chitosan, several challenges still need to be addressed. These include its mechanical properties, degradation rate, and immunogenicity. Researchers are actively investigating various strategies to enhance chitosan's mechanical strength, control its degradation rate, and minimize potential immune responses. Additionally, the incorporation of bioactive molecules and growth factors into chitosan-based constructs is being explored to further enhance their regenerative potential.

Conclusion:
Chitosan holds great potential as a versatile biomaterial in tissue engineering. Its unique properties, biocompatibility, and biodegradability make it suitable for various applications, including bone and cartilage tissue engineering. Ongoing research efforts aim to overcome the existing challenges and optimize chitosan-based constructs for improved tissue regeneration. As the field of tissue engineering continues to advance, chitosan is expected to play a crucial role in building a better tomorrow by enabling the development of innovative solutions for regenerative medicine.

Synthetic Biomaterials

In the field of tissue engineering, the development of synthetic biomaterials has revolutionized the way we approach the regeneration and repair of damaged tissues and organs. These materials, carefully designed to mimic the properties of natural tissues, have opened up new possibilities for medical interventions and have the potential to transform the future of healthcare.

Synthetic biomaterials are engineered materials that can be implanted into the human body to replace or repair damaged tissues. They are typically constructed from biocompatible polymers, ceramics, or metals, and are designed to promote cell adhesion, proliferation, and differentiation. These biomaterials serve as scaffolds that guide and support the growth of new tissue, helping the body to regenerate itself.

One of the key advantages of synthetic biomaterials is their versatility. Researchers can tailor their composition, physical properties, and surface characteristics to suit specific tissue engineering applications. This allows for the development of biomaterials with precise mechanical strength, porosity, and degradation rates, ensuring optimal integration with the surrounding tissues. Synthetic biomaterials also offer the advantage of being readily available in large quantities, making them a cost-effective option for medical treatments.

Synthetic biomaterials have been successfully used in a wide range of tissue engineering applications, including bone and cartilage regeneration, cardiovascular repair, and nerve regeneration. For example, biodegradable polymers such as poly(lactic acid) (PLA) and poly(glycolic acid) (PGA) have been used to create scaffolds for bone tissue engineering. These scaffolds provide a three-dimensional framework for bone cells to grow and regenerate, gradually degrading as new tissue forms.

In addition to their use as scaffolds, synthetic biomaterials can also be used to deliver therapeutic agents, such as growth factors or drugs, to the site of tissue damage. By incorporating these agents into the biomaterial, controlled release can be achieved, enhancing the healing process and reducing the risk of complications.

Despite the numerous advancements in synthetic biomaterials, challenges still remain. Ensuring long-term biocompatibility, minimizing the risk of infection, and improving the mechanical properties of these materials are ongoing areas of research. However, with continuous innovation and collaboration between materials scientists, engineers, and medical professionals, synthetic biomaterials hold immense promise for building a better tomorrow in tissue engineering and regenerative medicine.

In conclusion, synthetic biomaterials have emerged as a game-changer in tissue engineering, offering a viable solution for the repair and regeneration of damaged tissues and organs. With their versatile properties and ability to be tailored to specific applications, these materials have the potential to revolutionize the field of healthcare. By harnessing the power of synthetic biomaterials, we can pave the way for a brighter future in medical interventions and ultimately improve the lives of people around the world.

Polymers

Polymers: Building Blocks for Tissue Engineering

Introduction:

Polymers are an essential class of materials in the field of tissue engineering, offering a wide range of properties and functionalities that make them highly versatile for various applications. They have revolutionized the development of biomaterials and have played a crucial role in creating innovative solutions for tissue regeneration and repair. This subchapter explores the fascinating world of polymers, their unique characteristics, and their wide-ranging applications in tissue engineering.

Understanding Polymers:

Polymers are large molecules made up of repeating subunits called monomers. This structural arrangement allows for the formation of long chains or networks, providing the material with its distinctive properties. The flexibility of polymers allows for tailoring their mechanical, chemical, and biological properties to suit specific tissue engineering applications.

Polymer Types in Tissue Engineering:

There is a wide variety of polymers used in tissue engineering, each with its own set of advantages and limitations. Natural polymers, such as collagen, gelatin, and hyaluronic acid, offer excellent biocompatibility and bioactivity. Synthetic polymers, such as poly(lactic-co-glycolic acid) (PLGA), polyethylene glycol (PEG), and poly(caprolactone) (PCL), provide tunable mechanical properties and tailored degradation rates.

Applications of Polymers in Tissue Engineering:

Polymers serve as scaffolds for cell growth and tissue regeneration. They can be fabricated into 3D structures that mimic the native extracellular matrix, providing mechanical support and promoting cell adhesion, migration, and proliferation. Additionally, polymers can be functionalized with bioactive molecules, such as growth factors or peptides, to enhance cellular responses and guide tissue formation.

Polymeric Hydrogels:

Hydrogels are three-dimensional networks of cross-linked polymers that can retain a large amount of water. They are commonly used in tissue engineering due to their resemblance to soft tissues and their ability to deliver cells and bioactive molecules. Hydrogels can be engineered to possess specific mechanical and degradation properties, making them suitable for a wide range of tissue engineering applications, including wound healing, cartilage repair, and drug delivery.

Conclusion:

Polymers have revolutionized the field of tissue engineering, providing researchers and engineers with versatile materials to create advanced solutions for tissue repair and regeneration. The wide range of properties and functionalities offered by polymers make them invaluable in developing biomaterials that closely mimic the native environment of tissues. From natural polymers to synthetic ones, the versatility of polymers allows for tailoring materials to specific tissue engineering applications. With ongoing research and advancements in polymer science, we can look forward to a future where polymers continue to play a vital role in building a better tomorrow for tissue engineering.

Ceramics

Ceramics, in the context of materials science and engineering, are a class of inorganic materials that are known for their exceptional properties and wide range of applications. Derived from the Greek word "keramos," meaning pottery or clay, ceramics have been used by humans for thousands of years and continue to play a vital role in various industries and technologies today.

One of the defining characteristics of ceramics is their high melting points, which make them highly resistant to extreme temperatures. This property, coupled with their excellent mechanical strength and hardness, makes ceramics ideal for applications in high-temperature environments, such as aerospace and automotive industries. Ceramics are used as heat shields, engine components, and cutting tools, among others.

Another advantage of ceramics is their exceptional electrical properties. They are excellent electrical insulators, making them indispensable in electronics and telecommunications. Ceramics are used in the production of capacitors, resistors, and various other electronic components that require insulation and stability.

In recent years, ceramics have gained significant attention in the field of tissue engineering. The unique properties of ceramics, such as biocompatibility and bioactivity, make them excellent candidates for creating scaffolds for tissue regeneration. These scaffolds can provide structural support and promote cell growth, facilitating the regeneration of damaged tissues and organs. The use of ceramics in tissue engineering has shown great promise in applications such as bone and dental tissue regeneration.

Ceramics are also widely employed in the medical and dental fields. Dental ceramics, for instance, are used in the fabrication of dental crowns, bridges, and implants due to their biocompatibility and ability to mimic the natural appearance of teeth. In the medical field, ceramics are used in the production of implants, such as hip and knee replacements, due to their biocompatibility, strength, and resistance to wear.

In conclusion, ceramics are a versatile class of materials that find applications in a wide range of industries and technologies. Their exceptional properties, including high melting points, excellent mechanical strength, electrical insulation, and biocompatibility, make them invaluable in aerospace, automotive, electronics, tissue engineering, and medical fields. As research and development continue to advance, ceramics are likely to play an even more significant role in building a better tomorrow.

Metals

Metals are indispensable materials in various fields, including tissue engineering. Their unique properties make them ideal for tackling diverse challenges and creating innovative solutions. In this subchapter, we will explore the fascinating world of metals and their applications in tissue engineering, with a focus on their mechanical and biological properties.

One of the key advantages of metals is their exceptional strength and durability. This property allows them to provide structural support, making them indispensable for the construction of load-bearing implants and scaffolds. Titanium and its alloys, for instance, are widely used in orthopedic applications due to their excellent mechanical properties, corrosion resistance, and biocompatibility. These metals can integrate seamlessly with the surrounding bone tissue, promoting faster healing and recovery.

In addition to their mechanical properties, metals also possess unique biological characteristics that make them highly desirable for tissue engineering. Certain metals, such as magnesium, zinc, and iron, exhibit bioresorbability, meaning they can be gradually absorbed by the body over time. This property is particularly advantageous for temporary implants, as they can degrade naturally, eliminating the need for additional surgeries for their removal.

Metals can also be engineered to enhance their biological compatibility. Surface modifications, such as coatings or nanostructuring, can promote cell adhesion, proliferation, and differentiation. These modifications are crucial for successful integration of the implant with the surrounding tissues, ensuring long-term functionality.

Furthermore, metals can be combined with other materials to create hybrid composites with improved properties. For example, the combination of metals with ceramics or polymers can result in materials with enhanced mechanical strength, biocompatibility, and bioactivity. These composites are particularly beneficial for tissue engineering applications where both mechanical support and biological functionality are required.

In conclusion, metals play a vital role in tissue engineering, offering a wide range of applications and benefits. Their unique mechanical and biological properties make them indispensable for creating implants and scaffolds that can withstand the rigors of the human body while promoting tissue regeneration. By harnessing the power of metals, researchers and engineers in the field of tissue engineering are building a better tomorrow where innovative solutions are shaping the future of medicine.

Composites

In the world of materials science and engineering, composites play a crucial role in revolutionizing the field of tissue engineering. Composites, as the name suggests, are materials that consist of two or more distinct components combined together to create a new material with enhanced properties. These materials have become a cornerstone in the development of novel solutions for tissue engineering, offering a wide range of possibilities and applications.

Composites offer the ability to tailor the properties of a material to meet specific requirements, making them ideal for tissue engineering applications. By combining different materials such as polymers, ceramics, metals, and even natural fibers, researchers have been able to create composites with unique mechanical, chemical, and biological properties that mimic those found in natural tissues. This opens up a world of possibilities for creating scaffolds, implants, and other biomaterials that closely resemble the body's own tissues.

One example of a composite used in tissue engineering is the polymer-ceramic composite. By incorporating biodegradable polymers with bioactive ceramics, researchers have developed materials that not only provide structural support but also promote cell adhesion, proliferation, and differentiation. These composites can be used as scaffolds to guide tissue regeneration and promote the growth of new blood vessels.

Another exciting area of research in composites for tissue engineering is the use of natural fibers as reinforcement materials. Natural fibers such as silk, collagen, and cellulose have excellent biocompatibility and mechanical properties that make them ideal candidates for reinforcing polymer matrices. These natural fiber-reinforced composites can be used to create implants and tissue engineering scaffolds that closely resemble the mechanical properties of natural tissues, promoting better integration and healing.

Composites have also shown great promise in the field of drug delivery systems. By incorporating drug-loaded nanoparticles or microspheres into a composite material, researchers have been able to create materials that can release drugs in a controlled and sustained manner. This opens up possibilities for targeted drug delivery, minimizing side effects and improving the efficacy of treatments.

In conclusion, composites have revolutionized the field of tissue engineering, offering a versatile platform for the development of innovative biomaterials. By combining different materials, researchers can create composites with tailored properties that closely resemble those of natural tissues. These materials have the potential to advance the field of tissue engineering, leading to better treatments, improved patient outcomes, and a brighter future for regenerative medicine.

Biomimetic and Bioactive Materials

In recent years, there has been a growing interest in the field of tissue engineering, which aims to develop innovative solutions for repairing and regenerating damaged tissues and organs. One of the key aspects of tissue engineering is the development of materials that can mimic the natural environment of the body and promote the growth and function of cells. This subchapter explores the fascinating world of biomimetic and bioactive materials, which have the potential to revolutionize the field of tissue engineering.

Biomimetic materials are designed to replicate the structural and functional properties of natural tissues. By mimicking the architecture and composition of tissues such as bone, cartilage, and skin, these materials can provide a suitable environment for cell growth and tissue regeneration. For example, researchers have developed biomimetic scaffolds that mimic the structure of bone, with interconnected pores and channels that allow for the infiltration of cells and nutrients. These scaffolds can serve as a template for new bone formation, guiding the growth of cells and promoting tissue integration.

Bioactive materials, on the other hand, interact with the biological environment and stimulate specific cellular responses. These materials can release bioactive molecules, such as growth factors and cytokines, which play a crucial role in cell signaling and tissue regeneration. By incorporating bioactive molecules into scaffolds or coatings, researchers can enhance the healing process and improve tissue regeneration. For instance, bioactive materials can stimulate the recruitment of stem cells to the site of injury and promote their differentiation into specific cell types, such as osteoblasts or chondrocytes.

The development of biomimetic and bioactive materials requires a deep understanding of both materials science and biology. Researchers in the field of materials science and engineering play a crucial role in designing and fabricating these innovative materials. They explore various fabrication techniques, such as electrospinning, 3D printing, and self-assembly, to create biomimetic structures with precise control over their properties. Furthermore, they investigate the properties of bioactive molecules, such as their release kinetics and their effect on cell behavior.

In conclusion, biomimetic and bioactive materials hold great promise for the field of tissue engineering. By replicating the natural environment of the body and actively interacting with cells, these materials can promote tissue regeneration and improve patient outcomes. Researchers in the field of materials science and engineering continue to push the boundaries of innovation in this exciting area, bringing us closer to building a better tomorrow for tissue engineering.

Surface Modification Techniques

In the field of tissue engineering, the surface properties of biomaterials play a crucial role in determining their interactions with cells and tissues. Surface modification techniques have emerged as a powerful tool to tailor the surface properties of materials, allowing for improved biocompatibility, cell adhesion, and tissue integration. This subchapter explores various surface modification techniques employed in tissue engineering and their applications in building a better tomorrow.

One widely used surface modification technique is surface coating. This technique involves depositing a thin layer of biocompatible materials onto the surface of a biomaterial. These coatings can be designed to enhance cell adhesion, prevent bacterial colonization, or release bioactive molecules to regulate cellular behavior. Examples of commonly used coatings include hydroxyapatite, silk fibroin, and collagen. These coatings not only improve the biocompatibility of the material but also provide a suitable environment for cell attachment and proliferation.

Another surface modification technique is surface roughening. By altering the surface topography, the cell-material interaction can be enhanced. Micro- and nano-scale roughness can be created using various methods such as acid etching, plasma treatment, or laser ablation. This roughened surface promotes cell adhesion and migration, leading to improved tissue integration and regeneration. Research has shown that surface roughening techniques can significantly enhance the osteointegration of orthopedic implants and the vascularization of tissue-engineered constructs.

Surface functionalization is another important technique utilized in tissue engineering. This technique involves modifying the surface chemistry of biomaterials to promote specific cellular responses. One common method of surface functionalization is grafting bioactive molecules onto the material surface. For example, peptides, growth factors, or cytokines can be immobilized onto the material surface to enhance cell adhesion, proliferation, or differentiation. Additionally, surface functionalization can also be used to immobilize signaling molecules that regulate cellular behavior, such as cell adhesion peptides or anti-inflammatory agents.

Furthermore, surface patterning techniques have gained significant attention in tissue engineering. These techniques involve creating micro- or nano-scale patterns on the material surface to guide cell behavior. By controlling the spatial arrangement of surface features, cell alignment, migration, and tissue organization can be directed. Microcontact printing, photolithography, and electrospinning are some of the common techniques used for surface patterning.

In conclusion, surface modification techniques play a vital role in tissue engineering by tailoring the surface properties of biomaterials. These techniques allow for improved biocompatibility, cell adhesion, and tissue integration. Surface coating, roughening, functionalization, and patterning are some of the widely used techniques in this field. By employing these techniques, researchers and engineers are paving the way for the development of advanced biomaterials that can revolutionize the field of tissue engineering and contribute to building a better tomorrow for all.

Scaffolds and Tissue Matrices

In the field of tissue engineering, scaffolds and tissue matrices play a crucial role in the development of functional tissues and organs. These innovative materials serve as the structural support for cells to grow and differentiate, ultimately leading to the formation of new tissue. This subchapter aims to introduce the concept of scaffolds and tissue matrices, their importance in tissue engineering, and the advancements made in materials science and engineering.

Scaffolds are three-dimensional structures that mimic the extracellular matrix (ECM), the natural environment in which cells reside. They provide a framework for cells to adhere, proliferate, and eventually differentiate into functional tissue. The design of scaffolds involves careful considerations of their mechanical properties, biocompatibility, and degradation rate. Various materials such as polymers, ceramics, and hydrogels have been explored in the fabrication of scaffolds, each with unique advantages and limitations.

Tissue matrices, on the other hand, are decellularized tissue derived scaffolds that retain the composition and architecture of the natural ECM. These matrices preserve the intricate network of proteins, growth factors, and signaling molecules found in native tissues, providing an ideal microenvironment for cell attachment and tissue regeneration. They have shown great potential in promoting cell migration, angiogenesis, and tissue integration.

Materials science and engineering have contributed significantly to the development of scaffolds and tissue matrices. Advancements in biomaterials and fabrication techniques have enabled the creation of highly customizable and functional structures. Nanotechnology has further enhanced the mechanical and biological properties of scaffolds by incorporating nanoparticles and nanofibers. Researchers have also focused on developing bioactive materials that can release growth factors or drugs to guide cell behavior and tissue regeneration.

Furthermore, the characterization and evaluation of scaffolds and tissue matrices require interdisciplinary approaches. Techniques such as electron microscopy, mechanical testing, and molecular analysis help assess their structural integrity, biocompatibility, and bioactivity. This knowledge allows researchers to optimize scaffold design and fabrication processes, leading to improved tissue engineering strategies.

In conclusion, scaffolds and tissue matrices are essential elements in tissue engineering, providing the necessary support and cues for cell growth and tissue regeneration. Materials science and engineering have revolutionized the field by offering innovative biomaterials and fabrication techniques. With continued advancements, the development of functional tissues and organs for medical applications becomes increasingly promising.

Chapter 4: Materials for Medical Devices and Implants

Introduction to Medical Devices and Implants

In today's world, medical devices and implants play a crucial role in improving the quality of life for millions of people worldwide. From pacemakers and artificial joints to stents and prosthetic limbs, these innovative technologies have revolutionized the field of healthcare, offering new possibilities and solutions for patients of all ages and backgrounds. This subchapter aims to provide a comprehensive introduction to the fascinating world of medical devices and implants, exploring their importance, advancements, and impact on the field of materials science and engineering.

Medical devices are instruments, apparatus, implants, or machines used in the diagnosis, treatment, or prevention of diseases or other medical conditions. They can be as simple as a thermometer or as complex as a robotic surgical system. Implants, on the other hand, are devices that are surgically inserted into the body to replace a missing biological structure or support a damaged one. These can range from dental implants to artificial hips and even brain implants for deep brain stimulation.

Materials science and engineering have played a pivotal role in the development and improvement of medical devices and implants. The selection of appropriate materials is critical to ensure compatibility with the human body, durability, and functionality. Biocompatible materials such as metals, ceramics, polymers, and composites are extensively utilized due to their unique properties and ability to integrate seamlessly with the biological system.

Advancements in materials science have led to the development of innovative technologies that have significantly enhanced the performance and longevity of medical devices and implants. For instance, the introduction of shape memory alloys, such as Nitinol, has revolutionized the field of vascular interventions by enabling the creation of self-expanding stents that can restore blood flow with minimal invasive procedures. Similarly, the use of biodegradable polymers has opened new avenues for tissue engineering, allowing for the controlled release of drugs and growth factors to promote tissue regeneration.

In this subchapter, we will delve into the various types of medical devices and implants, including cardiovascular devices, orthopedic implants, dental devices, and neural interfaces. We will explore the materials used, their properties, and the challenges faced in their design and manufacturing. Moreover, we will discuss the regulatory framework governing medical devices and implants, ensuring their safety and efficacy.

Whether you are a materials science and engineering enthusiast or simply curious about the fascinating world of medical devices and implants, this subchapter will provide you with a solid foundation to understand the critical role these technologies play in improving healthcare outcomes and building a better tomorrow for all.

Metallic Materials for Medical Devices

In recent years, the field of materials science and engineering has made significant advancements in the development of metallic materials for medical devices. These materials have revolutionized the healthcare industry by providing innovative solutions for various medical applications. From prosthetic implants to surgical instruments, metallic materials have proven to be crucial in improving patient care and enhancing quality of life.

One of the primary advantages of metallic materials in medical devices is their exceptional mechanical properties. Metals such as titanium, stainless steel, and cobalt-chromium alloys exhibit high strength, superior wear resistance, and remarkable corrosion resistance. These properties make them ideal for load-bearing applications, where the devices are subjected to significant stress and strain. Metallic materials also possess the ability to withstand the harsh conditions within the human body, ensuring long-term performance and durability of medical implants.

Another important aspect of metallic materials is their biocompatibility. Extensive research and development efforts have been dedicated to enhancing the biocompatibility of these materials, ensuring they do not elicit adverse reactions within the body. Surface modifications, such as the application of biocompatible coatings and the use of bioactive materials, have significantly improved the integration of metallic implants with the surrounding tissues. This has resulted in reduced inflammation, accelerated healing, and enhanced biointegration, ultimately leading to better patient outcomes.

Furthermore, metallic materials offer versatility in design and manufacturing. Advanced techniques such as additive manufacturing, or 3D printing, have revolutionized the production of complex medical devices with intricate geometries. This allows for the customization of implants based on patient-specific needs, leading to improved fit, function, and overall success rates.

However, despite their numerous advantages, metallic materials are not without limitations. One major challenge is their inherent stiffness, which can lead to stress shielding and bone resorption. Researchers are actively working on developing new materials and composite structures that mimic the mechanical properties of natural tissues, thereby reducing these complications.

In conclusion, metallic materials have played a significant role in advancing the field of medical devices. Their exceptional mechanical properties, biocompatibility, and versatility have paved the way for innovative solutions in patient care. As materials science and engineering continue to evolve, the development of metallic materials for medical devices will undoubtedly contribute to building a better tomorrow in healthcare.

Stainless Steel

Stainless steel is a remarkable material that has revolutionized various industries, including the field of tissue engineering. In this subchapter, we will explore the unique properties of stainless steel and its applications in the context of building a better tomorrow for tissue engineering.

Stainless steel is an alloy composed primarily of iron, chromium, and nickel. Its corrosion-resistant nature makes it an ideal choice for medical implants and instruments. The addition of chromium forms a protective layer on the surface of the steel, preventing rust and corrosion. This property is crucial in tissue engineering, where biocompatible materials are necessary to ensure the success of implants and scaffolds.

One of the distinct advantages of stainless steel in tissue engineering lies in its mechanical properties. It exhibits high strength, durability, and resistance to wear and tear. These qualities make stainless steel an excellent candidate for load-bearing applications, such as orthopedic implants and prosthetics. Its ability to withstand mechanical stress and strain is crucial for long-term implant success and patient comfort.

Furthermore, stainless steel is highly versatile and can be easily fabricated into various shapes and forms. This versatility allows for the creation of customized implants tailored to meet individual patients' needs. For example, stainless steel can be machined into intricate shapes, ensuring a perfect fit for bone or tissue defects. Additionally, it can be easily sterilized, making it an excellent choice for medical instruments that require frequent cleaning and disinfection.

In tissue engineering, stainless steel finds applications in the development of scaffolds, which act as temporary support structures for tissue regeneration. These scaffolds provide a framework for cells to grow and differentiate, ultimately forming new tissues or organs. Stainless steel scaffolds offer mechanical stability and a controlled environment for cell growth, facilitating the regeneration process.

Moreover, stainless steel's biocompatibility and non-toxic nature make it an attractive material for tissue engineering. It does not elicit adverse immune responses or cause toxicity in the surrounding tissues. This biocompatibility ensures that the body can seamlessly integrate with stainless steel implants, promoting healing and long-term functionality.

In conclusion, stainless steel is a remarkable material that has found extensive applications in tissue engineering. Its unique combination of corrosion resistance, mechanical properties, versatility, and biocompatibility makes it an ideal choice for medical implants, instruments, and scaffolds. As researchers and engineers continue to explore the potential of materials for tissue engineering, stainless steel remains a crucial component in building a better tomorrow in the field of regenerative medicine.

Titanium Alloys

Titanium alloys have emerged as a critical group of materials in the field of tissue engineering due to their unique combination of mechanical properties, biocompatibility, and corrosion resistance. These alloys are widely used in orthopedic and dental implants, as well as in the fabrication of various medical devices.

One of the primary reasons for the popularity of titanium alloys is their exceptional biocompatibility. When in contact with living tissues, titanium alloys form a thin layer of titanium oxide on their surface, which promotes osseointegration - the direct integration of the implant with the surrounding bone tissue. This property ensures that the implants remain stable and firmly anchored in place, allowing for long-term success rates in clinical applications.

In addition to their biocompatibility, titanium alloys possess excellent mechanical properties. They have a high strength-to-weight ratio, which makes them ideal for load-bearing applications. This characteristic is especially important in orthopedic implants, where the material must withstand the forces exerted by the body. Titanium alloys are also known for their resistance to fatigue and wear, ensuring that the implants remain intact and functional for extended periods.

Corrosion resistance is another key attribute of titanium alloys. The formation of the protective titanium oxide layer on their surface makes them highly resistant to corrosion, even in aggressive physiological environments. This property is crucial for the long-term stability and performance of implants, as it prevents the release of harmful ions into the surrounding tissues.

Various types of titanium alloys are available, each with its own unique properties and applications. For example, commercially pure titanium (CP-Ti) is widely used due to its excellent biocompatibility and low modulus of elasticity, which closely matches that of bone. On the other hand, titanium alloys such as Ti-6Al-4V and Ti-6Al-7Nb contain additional elements to enhance their mechanical properties, making them suitable for load-bearing applications.

In conclusion, titanium alloys have revolutionized the field of tissue engineering. Their exceptional biocompatibility, mechanical properties, and corrosion resistance make them the material of choice for a wide range of medical applications. Whether it's an orthopedic implant or a dental prosthesis, titanium alloys offer the perfect combination of strength, stability, and biocompatibility required for successful tissue integration and long-term clinical outcomes.

Cobalt-Chromium Alloys

Cobalt-chromium alloys are an important class of materials in the field of materials science and engineering, especially in the context of tissue engineering. These alloys are widely used in the medical field due to their unique combination of mechanical strength, corrosion resistance, and biocompatibility. They have been extensively researched and developed for various applications in tissue engineering, making significant contributions to the field and paving the way for a better tomorrow.

One of the key advantages of cobalt-chromium alloys is their exceptional mechanical properties. They possess a high tensile strength, making them ideal for load-bearing applications. This attribute is particularly crucial in tissue engineering, where implants and scaffolds need to withstand the forces exerted by the surrounding tissues. The mechanical strength of these alloys ensures the longevity and durability of the engineered tissues, providing stability and support to the damaged or diseased areas.

Moreover, cobalt-chromium alloys exhibit excellent corrosion resistance, which is vital for maintaining the integrity of the implanted materials within the human body. The alloys form a protective oxide layer on their surface, preventing the release of harmful ions and minimizing the risk of corrosion. This characteristic ensures the long-term stability and functionality of the tissue-engineered constructs, minimizing the need for frequent replacements or revisions.

Biocompatibility is another critical feature of cobalt-chromium alloys. Extensive studies have demonstrated their compatibility with human tissues and cells, with minimal adverse reactions. This biocompatibility allows for proper integration of the implant or scaffold with the surrounding tissues, promoting tissue regeneration and healing. Furthermore, the materials' surface can be modified to enhance their interaction with biological entities, promoting cell adhesion, proliferation, and differentiation.

Cobalt-chromium alloys have been successfully employed in a wide range of tissue engineering applications, including orthopedics, dentistry, and cardiovascular interventions. They have been used to fabricate hip and knee implants, dental crowns and bridges, and stents, among others. The versatility of these alloys, coupled with their excellent properties, makes them a preferred choice for engineers and clinicians in the field.

In conclusion, cobalt-chromium alloys play a crucial role in the development of tissue engineering solutions. Their mechanical strength, corrosion resistance, and biocompatibility make them invaluable materials in the pursuit of building a better tomorrow. The continued research and advancements in cobalt-chromium alloys promise to revolutionize the field of tissue engineering, providing improved treatment options and enhancing the quality of life for patients worldwide.

Polymeric Materials for Medical Devices

In recent years, there has been a significant surge in the development of polymeric materials for medical devices. These materials have revolutionized the field of medicine, enabling the creation of advanced devices that are not only biocompatible but also possess tailored properties to enhance their performance. This subchapter aims to provide an overview of the key advancements in the field of polymeric materials for medical devices and their potential impact on the future of medicine.

Polymeric materials offer several advantages over traditional materials like metals and ceramics. Their flexibility, biocompatibility, and tunable properties make them ideal for a wide range of medical applications. One of the most significant breakthroughs in the field has been the development of biodegradable polymers. These polymers can be designed to degrade over time, allowing for the controlled release of drugs or the gradual regeneration of tissues.

Polymeric materials have found extensive use in implantable devices such as pacemakers, stents, and artificial joints. These devices require materials that can provide long-term stability within the body while minimizing the risk of adverse reactions. Polymeric materials have proven to be highly effective in meeting these requirements, offering excellent biocompatibility, corrosion resistance, and mechanical properties.

Furthermore, the versatility of polymeric materials allows for the incorporation of various functionalities to enhance device performance. For instance, surface modifications can be made to promote cell adhesion and tissue integration, reducing the risk of rejection and improving long-term device functionality. Additionally, the incorporation of nanoparticles or biomolecules within the polymer matrix can enable targeted drug delivery or enhance the antimicrobial properties of medical devices.

The field of polymeric materials for medical devices is continuously evolving, with ongoing research focused on improving their mechanical properties, biocompatibility, and overall performance. Future advancements may include the development of smart polymers that respond to external stimuli, such as temperature or pH changes, enabling dynamic control over device functionality. Furthermore, the integration of nanotechnology and biotechnology may lead to the creation of novel polymeric materials with unprecedented properties and capabilities.

In conclusion, the utilization of polymeric materials in medical devices has revolutionized the field of medicine. These materials offer several advantages, including biocompatibility, tunable properties, and the potential for controlled drug release. The continuous advancements in this field hold great promise for the development of innovative medical devices that can improve patient outcomes and contribute to building a better tomorrow in healthcare.

Polyethylene

Polyethylene: A Versatile Material for Tissue Engineering

Polyethylene is a widely used thermoplastic polymer that has found its applications in various fields, including tissue engineering. In this subchapter, we will explore the unique properties of polyethylene and its potential in the field of regenerative medicine. Whether you are a materials science and engineering enthusiast or someone interested in the future of healthcare, this subchapter will provide you with valuable insights into the role of polyethylene in tissue engineering.

Polyethylene is a synthetic polymer that can be produced with different molecular weights and densities, resulting in a wide range of material properties. Its high tensile strength, flexibility, and biocompatibility make it an ideal candidate for creating scaffolds in tissue engineering. Scaffolds are three-dimensional structures that mimic the extracellular matrix of natural tissues and provide a framework for cells to grow and regenerate damaged or diseased tissues.

One of the key advantages of polyethylene is its biocompatibility. It does not elicit an immune response or cause inflammation when implanted in the body, making it suitable for long-term applications. Additionally, polyethylene can be easily sterilized and processed into various forms, such as films, fibers, and porous scaffolds, which can be tailored to meet the specific requirements of different tissue types.

Polyethylene scaffolds can be fabricated using different techniques, including solvent casting, electrospinning, and 3D printing. These techniques allow for the precise control of scaffold structure, porosity, and mechanical properties, enabling the design of scaffolds that closely resemble the native tissue. By incorporating bioactive molecules, such as growth factors or drugs, into polyethylene scaffolds, researchers have been able to further enhance tissue regeneration.

Polyethylene has been successfully used in a variety of tissue engineering applications, including bone, cartilage, and vascular tissue regeneration. Its mechanical properties can be modulated to match those of the target tissue, providing the necessary support and mechanical cues for cell growth and differentiation. Moreover, polyethylene scaffolds have shown excellent biocompatibility and integration with the surrounding tissue, allowing for efficient tissue regeneration.

In conclusion, polyethylene is a versatile material with immense potential in tissue engineering. Its biocompatibility, mechanical properties, and processability make it an attractive choice for creating scaffolds that support tissue regeneration. As the field of tissue engineering advances, polyethylene will continue to play a crucial role in developing innovative solutions for a wide range of medical applications. Whether you are a materials science and engineering enthusiast or simply curious about the future of healthcare, exploring the potential of polyethylene in tissue engineering is a fascinating journey.

Silicone

Silicone is a versatile material that has found widespread applications in various fields, including tissue engineering. In this subchapter, we will explore the unique properties of silicone and its potential uses in the field of materials science and engineering.

Silicone is a synthetic polymer that is derived from silicon, a chemical element commonly found in sand and rocks. It is known for its exceptional stability, flexibility, and biocompatibility, making it an ideal choice for tissue engineering applications. Silicone can be easily molded into different shapes and sizes, allowing for the creation of customized implants, scaffolds, and prosthetics.

One of the key advantages of silicone is its biocompatibility. Unlike many other materials, silicone does not elicit a significant immune response when implanted into the body. This makes it an excellent material for medical devices, such as pacemakers, breast implants, and joint replacements. Additionally, silicone can be easily sterilized, ensuring aseptic conditions during implantation.

Silicone's flexibility is another desirable property that makes it suitable for tissue engineering. Its soft and pliable nature mimics the mechanical properties of natural tissues, providing a more natural feel and reducing the risk of implant failure. This flexibility also allows for easy integration with surrounding tissues, promoting tissue regeneration and healing.

In tissue engineering, silicone can be used to create scaffolds that provide structural support for cells to grow and differentiate. These scaffolds can be designed to mimic the architecture of specific tissues, facilitating the regeneration of damaged or diseased tissues. Silicone-based scaffolds can also be modified to release growth factors or drugs, enhancing the healing process and promoting tissue regeneration.

Silicone's stability is yet another advantage that makes it a valuable material in tissue engineering. It is resistant to degradation by heat, chemicals, and UV radiation, ensuring the longevity of implanted devices. This stability also allows for long-term monitoring and evaluation of tissue regeneration progress.

In conclusion, silicone is a remarkable material that offers numerous advantages for tissue engineering applications. Its biocompatibility, flexibility, and stability make it an excellent choice for the development of medical devices, implants, and scaffolds. As the field of materials science and engineering continues to advance, silicone will undoubtedly play a crucial role in building a better tomorrow in the realm of tissue engineering.

Polyurethane

Polyurethane is a versatile and widely used material in the field of tissue engineering. With its unique properties, it has revolutionized the way researchers approach the development of biomaterials for regenerative medicine. This subchapter aims to provide an overview of polyurethane and its applications in tissue engineering, addressing the audience of everyone interested in materials science and engineering.

Polyurethane is a synthetic polymer that can be tailored to exhibit a wide range of mechanical and chemical properties. This versatility makes it an excellent candidate for tissue engineering applications, where biomaterials must mimic the natural environment of cells and tissues. Polyurethanes can be designed to be biocompatible, biodegradable, and possess suitable mechanical strength, making them suitable for various tissue engineering applications.

One of the key advantages of polyurethane is its ability to be fabricated into different forms, such as films, foams, and scaffolds. These forms can be used to create structures that support cell growth and tissue regeneration. For example, polyurethane scaffolds can be engineered to mimic the extracellular matrix, providing a three-dimensional environment for cells to attach, proliferate, and differentiate.

Polyurethane is also known for its excellent mechanical properties, including high tensile strength and elasticity. This allows it to withstand the forces exerted by living tissues, making it suitable for applications such as artificial blood vessels and heart valves. Additionally, its elasticity can aid in the development of materials that can respond to dynamic physiological conditions, such as the expansion and contraction of blood vessels.

Moreover, polyurethane can be modified to enhance its bioactivity and promote specific cellular responses. For instance, bioactive molecules such as growth factors or drugs can be incorporated into polyurethane matrices to facilitate tissue regeneration or drug delivery. This versatility allows researchers to tailor polyurethane-based materials for specific tissue engineering applications, such as bone regeneration, skin grafting, or cartilage repair.

In conclusion, polyurethane is a remarkable material that has significantly contributed to the field of tissue engineering. Its unique properties, versatility, and ability to mimic the natural environment of cells make it an ideal choice for developing biomaterials that can support tissue regeneration. As the field of tissue engineering continues to evolve, polyurethane will likely play a crucial role in building a better tomorrow for regenerative medicine.

Ceramic Materials for Medical Devices

Ceramic materials have revolutionized the field of medical devices, offering unique properties that make them ideal for a wide range of applications. From dental implants to bone scaffolds, ceramics have proven to be a valuable tool in advancing healthcare technologies. In this subchapter, we will explore the various ceramic materials used in medical devices, their properties, and the impact they have on patient care.

One of the main advantages of ceramic materials is their biocompatibility. Unlike metals, ceramics do not cause adverse reactions within the body, making them an excellent choice for implantable medical devices. Additionally, ceramics are inert and do not corrode, ensuring the longevity of the device and minimizing the risk of infection or complications.

One commonly used ceramic material in medical devices is alumina (Al_2O_3). Alumina is known for its excellent mechanical properties, including high strength and wear resistance. These properties make it suitable for orthopedic implants, such as hip and knee replacements, where durability and load-bearing capabilities are crucial. Furthermore, alumina is biologically inert, reducing the risk of rejection and allowing for optimal tissue integration.

Another ceramic material gaining popularity in the medical field is zirconia (ZrO_2). Zirconia exhibits exceptional strength and fracture toughness, making it an ideal choice for dental implants. Its biocompatibility and tooth-colored appearance also contribute to its widespread use in cosmetic dentistry. Zirconia implants offer superior esthetics and longevity compared to traditional metal implants, providing patients with a more natural and durable solution.

In addition to alumina and zirconia, other ceramic materials, such as calcium phosphates and bioactive glasses, have shown promising results in tissue engineering applications. These materials can be used to fabricate scaffolds that mimic the structure of natural bone, promoting cell attachment and tissue regeneration. By providing a three-dimensional framework, ceramic scaffolds facilitate the growth of new tissue, making them invaluable in the field of regenerative medicine.

In conclusion, ceramic materials have revolutionized the medical device industry, offering a unique combination of biocompatibility, durability, and functional properties. From orthopedic implants to dental prosthetics, ceramics have played a significant role in improving patient care and quality of life. As researchers continue to explore new ceramic compositions and fabrication techniques, the potential for these materials in tissue engineering and regenerative medicine is limitless.

Alumina

Alumina, also known as aluminum oxide (Al_2O_3), is a versatile material that finds numerous applications in the field of materials science and engineering. This subchapter will delve into the properties, uses, and potential benefits of alumina in tissue engineering, aimed at an audience of diverse backgrounds.

Alumina is a ceramic material that exhibits exceptional mechanical strength, high melting point, and excellent resistance to chemical corrosion. These properties make it an ideal candidate for various tissue engineering applications, particularly in the development of biocompatible scaffolds. These scaffolds act as a framework for the growth and regeneration of tissues, providing mechanical support and guiding cell behavior.

One of the key advantages of alumina in tissue engineering is its biocompatibility. Extensive research has demonstrated that alumina does not elicit adverse reactions when in contact with living tissues. This makes it a safe and reliable material for use in implants, prosthetics, and other medical devices. Additionally, alumina's low friction coefficient and wear resistance make it suitable for applications in joint replacements, where it can improve the longevity and functionality of the implants.

Another significant benefit of alumina is its electrical insulation properties. This feature is particularly useful in applications such as neural tissue engineering, where electrical signaling plays a crucial role. By providing an electrically insulating environment, alumina can enhance the integration of implanted electrodes with neural tissues, enabling improved communication between prosthetic devices and the nervous system.

Moreover, alumina's chemical stability allows it to withstand harsh physiological conditions within the body. It can resist degradation caused by body fluids and enzymes, ensuring the longevity and structural integrity of tissue engineering constructs. This stability is especially important in long-term applications, where the materials must maintain their properties for extended periods.

In conclusion, alumina is a valuable material in tissue engineering due to its mechanical strength, biocompatibility, electrical insulation properties, and chemical stability. Its versatility and ability to adapt to various applications make it an essential tool in the development of better tissue engineering solutions. Whether it is used in scaffolds, implants, or prosthetics, alumina offers promising opportunities for building a better future in the field of tissue engineering.

Zirconia

Zirconia: A Versatile Material for the Future of Tissue Engineering

In the quest to build a better tomorrow for medical treatments and regenerative medicine, the field of tissue engineering plays a vital role. With the aim of creating functional tissues and organs, researchers and scientists are constantly exploring new materials that can mimic the complex structures and properties of the human body. Among these materials, zirconia has emerged as a versatile and promising candidate, holding immense potential in the field of tissue engineering.

Zirconia, also known as zirconium dioxide, is a ceramic material with unique properties that make it an excellent choice for various biomedical applications. Its exceptional biocompatibility, high mechanical strength, and resistance to wear and corrosion make it an ideal material for use in tissue engineering scaffolds, implants, and other biomedical devices.

One of the key advantages of zirconia is its biocompatibility, meaning it can interact with living tissues without causing any adverse reactions. This property is of utmost importance when designing materials for tissue engineering, as it ensures the successful integration of the implant or scaffold with the surrounding tissues. Zirconia's biocompatibility allows for better cell adhesion, proliferation, and differentiation, enabling the formation of functional tissues.

Furthermore, zirconia's mechanical strength is comparable to that of human bone, making it an excellent substitute material for bone grafts and implants. Its high fracture toughness ensures the stability and durability of implants, reducing the risk of failure. This property is particularly crucial in load-bearing applications, where the material needs to withstand the mechanical forces exerted by the body.

In addition to its mechanical properties, zirconia also possesses excellent wear resistance and corrosion resistance. This makes it an ideal material choice for dental implants, as it can withstand the harsh environment of the oral cavity and resist degradation over time. Zirconia-based dental implants have gained significant popularity in recent years due to their long-term stability and aesthetic appeal.

Moreover, zirconia can be fabricated into highly porous scaffolds with interconnected pore networks, allowing for efficient nutrient and waste exchange within the tissue-engineered constructs. These scaffolds provide a three-dimensional structure that supports cell growth, proliferation, and tissue formation.

In conclusion, zirconia represents a promising material for the future of tissue engineering. Its exceptional biocompatibility, mechanical strength, and resistance to wear and corrosion make it an ideal choice for various biomedical applications. As researchers continue to explore its potential, zirconia holds the key to building a better tomorrow for regenerative medicine, offering hope for improved treatments and enhanced quality of life for patients worldwide.

Note: The content provided is within the word limit specified, but it is important to note that a comprehensive discussion on zirconia and its applications in tissue engineering would require more in-depth information and may exceed the given word count.

Hydroxyapatite

Hydroxyapatite: The Building Block of Tissue Engineering

Hydroxyapatite, the mineral form of calcium phosphate, is a key component in the field of tissue engineering, revolutionizing the way we approach the regeneration and repair of damaged tissues and organs. In this subchapter, we will explore the incredible properties of hydroxyapatite and its applications in the realm of materials science and engineering.

Hydroxyapatite, with its chemical formula $Ca_{10}(PO_4)_6(OH)_2$, closely resembles the structure of natural bone. This similarity makes it an ideal material for bone grafts, dental implants, and other orthopedic applications. When implanted in the human body, hydroxyapatite provides a scaffold for new bone tissue to grow, eventually integrating with the surrounding natural bone. Its biocompatibility ensures that it is well-tolerated by the body, minimizing the risk of rejection or adverse reactions.

One of the most remarkable qualities of hydroxyapatite is its ability to promote osteointegration, the process by which bone cells attach to and grow on the surface of an implant. This property is attributed to the similarity in crystal structure between hydroxyapatite and the mineral phase of bone. By mimicking the natural environment, hydroxyapatite encourages the formation of strong bonds between the implant and the surrounding bone, resulting in improved functionality and longevity of the implant.

Furthermore, hydroxyapatite can be synthesized in various forms, such as powders, coatings, and porous scaffolds, allowing for versatility in its applications. These forms can be tailored to specific requirements, such as controlling porosity, surface area, or mechanical strength, depending on the intended use. Additionally, hydroxyapatite can be combined with other biomaterials, such as polymers or metals, to enhance its mechanical properties and expand its range of applications.

In the field of dental engineering, hydroxyapatite plays a crucial role in the development of bioactive tooth restorations. By incorporating hydroxyapatite-based materials into dental composites, researchers aim to promote the regeneration of dentin, enamel, and other tooth tissues, ultimately leading to more durable and natural-looking dental restorations.

In conclusion, hydroxyapatite stands as a remarkable material in the realm of tissue engineering, offering a promising solution for the regeneration and repair of damaged tissues and organs. Its biocompatibility, osteointegration-promoting properties, and versatility make it a valuable building block for the future of materials science and engineering. With ongoing research and advancements, hydroxyapatite is poised to contribute significantly to the development of better, safer, and more effective tissue engineering solutions for a wide range of medical applications.

Chapter 5: Engineering Approaches in Tissue Engineering

Scaffold Fabrication Techniques

In the field of tissue engineering, scaffold fabrication techniques play a crucial role in creating three-dimensional structures that mimic the natural environment of cells and tissues. These scaffolds provide support, guidance, and a suitable environment for cells to grow and differentiate, ultimately leading to the regeneration of functional tissues. This subchapter will delve into various scaffold fabrication techniques used in tissue engineering, highlighting their advantages and limitations.

One of the commonly employed techniques is electrospinning. Electrospinning involves the use of an electric field to generate ultrafine fibers from a polymer solution or melt. This technique allows for the production of scaffolds with high porosity, large surface area, and controllable fiber diameter. The resulting nanofibrous structure closely resembles the extracellular matrix, promoting cell adhesion, proliferation, and tissue regeneration.

Another popular technique is 3D bioprinting, which enables the precise deposition of cells and biomaterials in a layer-by-layer manner to create complex three-dimensional structures. This technique offers great versatility in terms of scaffold design and customization, allowing for the incorporation of multiple cell types, growth factors, and bioactive molecules. However, challenges such as the selection of suitable bioinks and maintaining cell viability during the printing process need to be addressed for successful tissue regeneration.

In addition to these techniques, other scaffold fabrication methods include freeze-drying, solvent casting, and particulate leaching. Freeze-drying involves freezing a polymer solution followed by sublimation to remove the solvent, leaving behind a porous scaffold structure. Solvent casting entails the pouring of a polymer solution into a mold, which is then evaporated to create a solid scaffold. Particulate leaching involves the addition of sacrificial particles to a polymer solution, which are subsequently dissolved to create interconnected pores within the scaffold.

Each scaffold fabrication technique has its own advantages and limitations, making it essential to choose the most suitable method based on the requirements of the desired tissue. Factors such as mechanical properties, pore size, surface characteristics, and biocompatibility need to be carefully considered during scaffold fabrication to ensure successful tissue regeneration.

By understanding and utilizing various scaffold fabrication techniques, researchers and engineers in the field of tissue engineering can continue to advance the development of biomimetic scaffolds that facilitate tissue regeneration. These techniques hold great potential in building a better tomorrow by addressing the growing need for functional tissue replacements and therapies in various medical applications.

Note: The content provided above is a generated sample for the given title and audience. It is advised to proofread and modify the content to fit the specific requirements and tone of your book.

Salt Leaching

Salt leaching is a widely used technique in the field of materials science and engineering, particularly in the area of tissue engineering. This process involves the removal of salts from a material, leaving behind a porous structure that is highly suitable for tissue regeneration and scaffold development.

The concept behind salt leaching is quite simple. A salt, such as sodium chloride, is mixed with a polymer or other material of interest. This mixture is then shaped into the desired form, such as a scaffold or implant. The salt particles act as porogens, creating void spaces within the material when dissolved or removed. These void spaces are crucial for cell infiltration and nutrient transport, making salt leaching an essential step in the fabrication of tissue-engineered constructs.

The salt leaching process typically involves three main steps: fabrication, leaching, and drying. During the fabrication step, the polymer and salt are mixed together and shaped into the desired form using various techniques such as molding or 3D printing. The leaching step involves immersing the fabricated construct in a solvent, such as water, that can dissolve the salt particles. As the salt dissolves, the void spaces are created within the material. Finally, the construct is dried to remove any remaining solvent, resulting in a porous structure ready for tissue engineering applications.

Salt leaching offers several advantages for tissue engineering. Firstly, it allows for the creation of highly porous structures with interconnected pores, mimicking the natural extracellular matrix found in tissues. This enhances cell infiltration and nutrient diffusion, promoting tissue regeneration. Additionally, the technique is versatile and can be used with a wide range of materials, including polymers, ceramics, and composites. This flexibility allows researchers to tailor the properties of the scaffold to meet specific tissue engineering requirements.

However, salt leaching also presents some challenges. One of the main concerns is the potential loss of mechanical strength in the material due to the creation of void spaces. This issue can be addressed by incorporating additives or reinforcements to enhance the mechanical properties of the scaffold. Another challenge is the control of pore size and porosity, as these factors can greatly influence cell behavior and tissue formation. Advanced fabrication techniques and precise control over the leaching process are essential for achieving the desired pore structure.

In conclusion, salt leaching is a valuable technique in the field of tissue engineering, offering a way to create porous structures that promote cell infiltration and tissue regeneration. By understanding the principles and challenges associated with salt leaching, researchers can develop improved materials for tissue engineering, bringing us closer to a better tomorrow in the field of regenerative medicine.

Electrospinning

Electrospinning is a versatile technique that holds immense potential in the field of materials science and engineering, particularly in tissue engineering applications. This subchapter aims to provide an overview of electrospinning and its role in building a better tomorrow for tissue engineering.

Electrospinning is a process that involves the creation of ultrafine fibers by subjecting a polymer solution or melt to an electric field. The process utilizes the surface tension of the polymer solution and the repulsion between the like charges to create a jet of polymer solution, which is then solidified into fibers upon reaching a collector. These fibers possess unique properties such as high surface area-to-volume ratio, tunable mechanical properties, and the ability to mimic the extracellular matrix (ECM) of natural tissues.

One of the major advantages of electrospinning is its ability to fabricate scaffolds with nanometer-scale fibers that can mimic the native architecture of various tissues. This feature is crucial for tissue engineering applications as it allows for better cell adhesion, proliferation, and differentiation. The electrospun scaffolds can be designed to closely resemble the ECM of specific tissues, providing an ideal microenvironment for cell growth and tissue regeneration.

Moreover, electrospinning allows for the incorporation of various bioactive molecules, such as growth factors and drugs, into the polymer solution. These molecules can be released in a controlled manner, promoting cell behavior and tissue regeneration. This controlled release feature is particularly beneficial for tissue engineering applications where timed and localized delivery of bioactive molecules is crucial for successful tissue regeneration.

In addition to its advantages in tissue engineering, electrospinning is a simple and cost-effective technique that can be easily scaled up for industrial production. This makes it highly attractive for commercial applications and further research and development in the materials science and engineering field.

Overall, electrospinning holds great promise for tissue engineering applications and is revolutionizing the way we approach tissue regeneration. By utilizing this technique to fabricate biomimetic scaffolds with tailored properties, researchers and scientists are paving the way for a better tomorrow in the field of materials science and engineering.

3D Printing

In recent years, 3D printing has emerged as a groundbreaking technology with the potential to revolutionize various industries, including tissue engineering. This subchapter aims to provide an overview of 3D printing techniques and their applications in the field of materials science and engineering, specifically in tissue engineering.

3D printing, also known as additive manufacturing, is a process that allows for the creation of three-dimensional objects layer by layer, based on digital designs. Unlike traditional manufacturing methods that involve subtractive processes, such as cutting or drilling, 3D printing adds material to build the desired structure. This unique approach offers unparalleled design freedom and customization capabilities.

In tissue engineering, 3D printing has opened up new possibilities for fabricating complex structures that mimic the architecture of natural tissues and organs. By depositing bioinks, which are materials composed of living cells and biomaterials, layer by layer, researchers can create tissue-like structures that have the potential to integrate seamlessly with the human body.

One of the key advantages of 3D printing in tissue engineering is the ability to create patient-specific implants or scaffolds. By utilizing patient-specific data, such as medical imaging scans, researchers can design and fabricate implants that perfectly fit the individual's anatomy. This personalized approach not only improves the implant's functionality but also enhances patient outcomes and reduces the risk of complications.

Moreover, 3D printing enables the fabrication of complex structures with precisely controlled microarchitectures. This control over the internal structure of tissue-engineered constructs can influence cellular behavior, including cell adhesion, proliferation, and differentiation. By mimicking the natural tissue microenvironment, 3D-printed scaffolds can promote tissue regeneration and guide the growth of new cells.

In addition to tissue engineering, 3D printing has found applications in drug delivery systems, medical devices, and prosthetics. Its versatility and adaptability make it a promising tool for advancing personalized medicine and improving patient care.

In conclusion, 3D printing holds immense potential in the field of tissue engineering and materials science and engineering as a whole. Its ability to create complex structures, customize designs, and integrate living cells makes it a valuable tool for building a better tomorrow in healthcare. As this technology continues to evolve, it is crucial for researchers, engineers, and medical professionals to embrace and explore its possibilities to unlock new frontiers in tissue engineering and ultimately improve the lives of patients worldwide.

Cell Seeding and Culturing Techniques

In tissue engineering, the successful integration of cells with biomaterials is a critical step towards building functional tissue constructs. The process of cell seeding and culturing involves carefully manipulating cells onto biomaterial scaffolds and providing them with an environment that promotes their growth and differentiation. This subchapter explores various techniques used in cell seeding and culturing, highlighting their significance in the field of tissue engineering.

One widely used technique for cell seeding is direct cell seeding, where cells are simply pipetted onto the surface of a biomaterial scaffold. This method allows for easy cell distribution and attachment, but it often results in uneven cell distribution and limited cell penetration into the scaffold. To address these limitations, researchers have developed alternative techniques such as cell spraying and cell printing. Cell spraying involves the use of a high-pressure nozzle to disperse cells onto the scaffold, promoting more uniform cell distribution. On the other hand, cell printing utilizes specialized printers to precisely place cells onto the scaffold in a controlled manner, enabling the creation of complex tissue architectures.

Once the cells are seeded onto the scaffold, they need to be cultured in an environment that supports their growth and functionality. This typically involves providing the cells with a culture medium that contains essential nutrients, growth factors, and signaling molecules. The culture medium also needs to be maintained at optimal conditions, including temperature, pH, and oxygenation, to promote cell viability and proliferation.

In addition to the culture medium, techniques such as bioreactors and perfusion systems have been developed to enhance cell culturing. Bioreactors provide a controlled environment for cells by mimicking the mechanical forces and biochemical cues present in native tissues. They can be designed to apply mechanical stimulation, such as cyclic stretching or compression, which can influence cell behavior and tissue development. Perfused systems, on the other hand, involve the continuous flow of culture medium through the scaffold, facilitating nutrient delivery and waste removal.

Overall, cell seeding and culturing techniques play a crucial role in tissue engineering by ensuring the successful integration and growth of cells within biomaterial scaffolds. These techniques are continually evolving and improving, paving the way for the development of more sophisticated tissue constructs that closely resemble native tissues. By understanding and utilizing these techniques, researchers and engineers in the field of materials science and engineering can contribute to building a better tomorrow through advancements in tissue engineering.

Static Seeding

In the realm of tissue engineering, one of the key challenges is to develop strategies that effectively promote cell attachment and proliferation on scaffolds. Static seeding is a technique commonly employed to address this issue, playing a crucial role in the success of tissue engineering approaches.

Static seeding involves the controlled placement of cells onto a scaffold in a stationary or static culture environment. This technique allows for a more uniform distribution of cells, ensuring their attachment and subsequent growth on the scaffold. By carefully manipulating the seeding conditions, researchers can optimize cell-scaffold interactions, thereby enhancing the overall success of tissue engineering strategies.

A critical aspect of static seeding is the choice of scaffold material. Materials scientists and engineers play a pivotal role in developing and designing scaffolds that possess the necessary characteristics to support cell attachment and growth. These materials must be biocompatible, providing an environment conducive to cellular adhesion and proliferation. Additionally, the scaffold should possess appropriate mechanical properties to mimic the natural extracellular matrix, ensuring the development of functional tissues.

The success of static seeding also relies on the appropriate cell source. Different tissues require specific cell types, and researchers need to carefully select and isolate the desired cells for seeding. These cells must maintain their viability and functionality throughout the seeding process to ensure successful tissue development.

Furthermore, the technique of static seeding allows for the introduction of multiple cell types onto a scaffold. This concept is particularly relevant in the development of complex tissues and organs, where the presence of different cell populations is crucial. By incorporating various cell types, researchers can create a microenvironment that promotes cellular communication and tissue integration, ultimately leading to the formation of functional and physiologically relevant tissues.

Static seeding is a versatile technique that can be applied to a wide range of tissue engineering applications. From the regeneration of bone and cartilage to the development of vascularized tissues and organs, static seeding provides a valuable tool in the construction of engineered tissues. The ability to control cell placement and distribution on scaffolds is fundamental to the success of tissue engineering approaches, and static seeding offers a means to achieve this control.

In conclusion, static seeding is a vital technique in tissue engineering, allowing for the controlled placement and distribution of cells on scaffolds. Materials scientists and engineers play a key role in developing suitable scaffold materials, while researchers carefully select and isolate appropriate cell sources. The technique enables the creation of functional tissues by promoting cellular attachment, proliferation, and communication. Static seeding holds immense potential for advancing the field of tissue engineering and offers hope for building a better tomorrow in the realm of regenerative medicine.

Perfusion Bioreactors

Perfusion bioreactors are an integral component of tissue engineering, playing a crucial role in the development and production of functional tissues. These bioreactors provide a controlled environment for the cultivation of cells, enabling the optimization of tissue growth and development.

In tissue engineering, the ultimate goal is to create tissues and organs that can replace or repair damaged or diseased ones. To achieve this, it is essential to mimic the natural physiological conditions in which cells reside and grow. Perfusion bioreactors allow researchers to recreate the dynamic microenvironment that cells experience in the human body, including the supply of nutrients, oxygen, and the removal of waste products.

The concept of perfusion involves the continuous flow of culture media through a porous scaffold that supports the cells. The scaffold serves as a three-dimensional framework, providing mechanical support and guiding cell growth. The perfusion of media through the scaffold ensures the delivery of nutrients and oxygen to the cells, while waste products are efficiently removed. This constant exchange of fluids enhances cell viability, proliferation, and differentiation, leading to the formation of functional tissues.

Materials science and engineering play a crucial role in the design and fabrication of perfusion bioreactors. The choice of materials for the scaffold and bioreactor components is critical to ensure biocompatibility, mechanical stability, and the ability to support cell growth. Researchers have explored a wide range of materials, including natural polymers, synthetic polymers, and hybrid materials, to develop scaffolds with optimal properties for tissue engineering applications.

The design of perfusion bioreactors also involves considerations such as flow rate, shear stress, and nutrient gradients. These parameters need to be carefully controlled to create an environment that promotes tissue formation and avoids detrimental effects on cell viability and function. Advances in computational modeling and simulation techniques have greatly aided in the optimization and understanding of these design parameters.

Perfusion bioreactors have revolutionized tissue engineering, enabling the production of functional tissues that closely resemble native tissues. They have found applications in various fields, including bone regeneration, cartilage repair, and organ transplantation. The continuous advancements in materials science and engineering are driving the development of more sophisticated bioreactors that can mimic the complex microenvironments found in different tissues. These advancements hold great promise for the future of tissue engineering, paving the way for the creation of better and more efficient therapies for a wide range of diseases and injuries.

In conclusion, perfusion bioreactors are a vital tool in tissue engineering, allowing researchers to create functional tissues by mimicking the natural physiological conditions in the human body. Materials science and engineering play a significant role in the design and fabrication of these bioreactors, ensuring biocompatibility, mechanical stability, and optimal cell growth. The continuous advancements in this field hold great promise for the development of better treatments and therapies, benefiting a wide range of medical applications.

Co-culture Techniques

In the field of tissue engineering, the development of effective techniques that can mimic the complex microenvironment of living tissues is crucial for the successful regeneration and repair of damaged or diseased tissues. One such technique that has gained significant attention in recent years is co-culture.

Co-culture involves the simultaneous cultivation of multiple cell types in a controlled environment, allowing for the study of cellular interactions, communication, and tissue development. By combining different cell types, researchers are able to recreate the complexity and functionality of native tissues, ultimately leading to more successful tissue engineering strategies.

One of the main advantages of co-culture techniques is the ability to recreate the dynamic cellular interactions that occur in vivo. In native tissues, cells communicate with each other through various signaling pathways, influencing their behavior and function. By co-culturing different cell types, researchers can investigate these interactions and understand how they contribute to tissue development and regeneration.

Moreover, co-culture techniques enable the creation of tissue constructs that closely resemble the native tissue architecture. For example, in bone tissue engineering, co-culturing osteoblasts and endothelial cells can facilitate the formation of blood vessels within the engineered bone, mimicking the vascularization process in natural bone. This vascular network is essential for the survival and function of the engineered tissue, as it allows the transport of nutrients and oxygen.

In addition to mimicking native tissues, co-culture techniques can also be used to study disease progression and develop new therapeutic approaches. By co-culturing healthy and diseased cells, researchers can investigate the underlying mechanisms of disease, test potential drug candidates, and develop personalized medicine strategies.

However, co-culture techniques also present challenges. The selection of appropriate cell types, their ratios, and the culture conditions must be carefully considered to achieve successful co-cultures. Additionally, the development of biomaterial scaffolds that support the growth and interaction of multiple cell types is crucial for the creation of functional tissue constructs.

In conclusion, co-culture techniques have revolutionized the field of tissue engineering by providing a platform to study cellular interactions, recreate native tissue architecture, and develop new therapeutic strategies. By combining different cell types, researchers can gain valuable insights into tissue development, disease progression, and ultimately, build a better tomorrow for patients in need of tissue regeneration and repair.

(Note: This content has been written for an audience of "EVERY ONE" interested in the niches of "Materials Science and Engineering".)

Tissue Engineering Strategies

In recent years, tissue engineering has emerged as a promising field that holds the potential to revolutionize the medical industry. By combining principles of materials science and engineering with biological knowledge, scientists and researchers are paving the way for building a better tomorrow in healthcare. This subchapter will delve into the various tissue engineering strategies that are being explored, highlighting their significance and potential impact.

One of the key strategies in tissue engineering is the use of biomaterials. These materials act as scaffolds, providing a three-dimensional structure that supports the growth and development of cells. Biomaterials can be synthetic or natural, and their selection depends on the specific tissue being engineered. Synthetic materials offer advantages such as controlled degradation rates and mechanical properties, while natural materials like collagen and hyaluronic acid provide a more biocompatible environment. The choice of biomaterial is crucial as it directly influences the success of tissue regeneration.

Another important strategy is the incorporation of growth factors and cytokines. These signaling molecules play a vital role in cell proliferation, migration, and differentiation. By incorporating these factors into the scaffold, tissue engineers can create a microenvironment that mimics the natural tissue regeneration process. The controlled release of growth factors ensures that cells receive the necessary cues to promote tissue formation and repair.

Cell sourcing is an essential aspect of tissue engineering. Stem cells, in particular, hold immense potential due to their ability to differentiate into various cell types. Embryonic stem cells, induced pluripotent stem cells, and adult stem cells are among the different cell sources being explored. Each cell source has its advantages and limitations, and researchers are working towards optimizing their use in tissue engineering applications.

Bioprinting, a cutting-edge technology, has gained traction in tissue engineering. It enables the precise deposition of cells and biomaterials in a layer-by-layer fashion, resulting in the creation of complex tissue constructs. This approach allows for the fabrication of tissues with intricate geometries and organized cell patterns, mimicking native tissues more closely.

The success of tissue engineering strategies heavily relies on understanding the interactions between cells and materials. Researchers are investigating cell-material interactions at the molecular level to design materials that promote cell adhesion, proliferation, and differentiation. Surface modifications, such as the incorporation of bioactive molecules and nanostructured features, are being explored to enhance cell material interactions and ultimately improve tissue regeneration outcomes.

The field of tissue engineering holds great promise for the future of healthcare. By combining materials science and engineering principles with biological knowledge, researchers are developing innovative strategies to regenerate damaged tissues and organs. These strategies, ranging from biomaterial selection to bioprinting, aim to create functional tissue constructs that can restore and improve the quality of life for countless individuals. As materials scientists and engineers, it is our duty to contribute to this exciting field and build a better tomorrow for everyone.

In vitro Engineering

In the field of tissue engineering, the development of innovative materials plays a crucial role in creating advanced biomedical devices and therapies. One such technique that has emerged as a promising solution is in vitro engineering. In this subchapter, we will explore the concept of in vitro engineering and its potential to revolutionize the field of materials science and engineering.

In vitro engineering involves the fabrication of tissues and organs outside the human body using a combination of biomaterials and living cells. Unlike traditional tissue engineering methods that rely on in vivo techniques, in vitro engineering offers several advantages. It enables researchers to have precise control over the fabrication process, creating tissues with specific characteristics tailored to the patient's needs.

The cornerstone of in vitro engineering is the selection and design of appropriate biomaterials. These materials should possess a unique combination of biocompatibility, mechanical properties, and bioactivity to support cell growth and tissue development. Materials scientists and engineers work together to develop novel biomaterials that can mimic the native extracellular matrix, providing a suitable microenvironment for cell adhesion, proliferation, and differentiation.

One of the key challenges in in vitro engineering is the successful integration of cells into the biomaterial scaffold. Researchers have devised various techniques to achieve this, including cell seeding, bioreactors, and microfluidic systems. These methods ensure uniform cell distribution and promote cell viability, ultimately leading to the formation of functional tissues.

The applications of in vitro engineering are wide-ranging and transformative. It has the potential to revolutionize the field of regenerative medicine by providing solutions for organ transplantation, wound healing, and tissue repair. Additionally, in vitro engineering can be used to develop personalized medicine approaches, where tissues are engineered to match a patient's specific needs, reducing the risk of rejection and improving treatment outcomes.

Furthermore, in vitro engineering allows for the study of disease mechanisms and drug testing in a controlled environment. Researchers can create disease models using patient-specific cells, enabling them to gain insights into disease progression and develop targeted therapies.

In conclusion, in vitro engineering is a cutting-edge technique within the field of tissue engineering. It offers immense potential for the development of advanced biomedical devices and therapies. With the collaborative efforts of materials scientists and engineers, in vitro engineering holds the promise of building a better tomorrow by revolutionizing the way we approach tissue regeneration and personalized medicine.

In vivo Engineering

In the field of tissue engineering, researchers are constantly striving to develop innovative and effective strategies to repair and regenerate damaged or diseased tissues and organs. One such approach that holds tremendous promise is in vivo engineering. This subchapter delves into the concept of in vivo engineering, its methodologies, and the potential it holds for building a better tomorrow in the field of materials science and engineering.

In vivo engineering refers to the development and application of biomaterials and tissue engineering strategies directly within the living organism. Unlike traditional tissue engineering techniques that involve the fabrication of tissues in the laboratory and subsequent implantation, in vivo engineering takes a more dynamic and integrated approach. By utilizing the body's own regenerative capacity, in vivo engineering aims to promote the repair and regeneration of tissues by guiding and supporting the natural healing processes.

One of the key advantages of in vivo engineering is its ability to harness the body's innate healing mechanisms. By providing a supportive environment and delivering the necessary cues, such as growth factors and scaffolds, in vivo engineering can enhance the regenerative potential of the body. This approach minimizes the need for invasive surgeries and reduces the risk of rejection, making it an attractive option for patients.

The subchapter further explores the various methodologies employed in in vivo engineering, including the use of biomaterials, growth factors, and stem cells. It discusses the design considerations for developing biomaterials that can integrate seamlessly into the host tissue, promoting cell adhesion, proliferation, and differentiation. The role of growth factors in stimulating tissue regeneration and the potential of stem cells in replenishing damaged or diseased tissues are also explored in detail.

Furthermore, the subchapter sheds light on the challenges and future directions of in vivo engineering. It highlights the need for bioactive materials with improved mechanical properties and biocompatibility, as well as the importance of understanding the host response to the implanted materials. Additionally, the potential applications of in vivo engineering beyond tissue regeneration, such as drug delivery and disease modeling, are also discussed.

In conclusion, in vivo engineering represents a promising approach in the field of tissue engineering. By working in harmony with the body's healing processes, it offers exciting possibilities for repairing and regenerating damaged tissues and organs. This subchapter serves as an informative guide for researchers, clinicians, and anyone interested in the advancements in materials science and engineering, highlighting the potential of in vivo engineering in building a better tomorrow for healthcare.

Ex vivo Engineering

Ex vivo engineering is a groundbreaking field within tissue engineering that holds immense promise for building a better tomorrow in the realm of regenerative medicine. In this subchapter, we will delve into the fascinating world of ex vivo engineering, exploring its principles, applications, and the role of materials science and engineering in this innovative area of research.

Ex vivo engineering refers to the manipulation and modification of cells, tissues, or organs outside the living organism to enhance their functionality or address specific medical conditions. Unlike in vivo engineering, which involves directly altering tissues within the body, ex vivo engineering offers several advantages, including better control over the environment, ease of manipulation, and the ability to perform complex procedures that may not be feasible in vivo.

One of the key aspects of ex vivo engineering is the use of advanced materials that can mimic the properties of native tissues and provide a suitable environment for cell growth and differentiation. Materials science and engineering play a pivotal role in designing and fabricating these biomaterials, which can range from natural substances like collagen and hyaluronic acid to synthetic polymers and biocompatible metals.

These materials must possess specific characteristics such as biocompatibility, mechanical strength, and the ability to support cell adhesion and proliferation. Researchers in the field of materials science and engineering are constantly exploring novel materials and fabrication techniques to create scaffolds, hydrogels, and microenvironments that closely resemble the natural extracellular matrix and promote tissue regeneration.

Ex vivo engineering has tremendous applications across various medical fields, including organ transplantation, tissue repair, and drug discovery. By cultivating and modifying cells outside the body, scientists can create functional tissues or organs that can be transplanted to replace damaged or diseased ones. This approach holds great potential for addressing the shortage of donor organs and improving the success rates of transplantation procedures.

Furthermore, ex vivo engineering enables researchers to develop personalized medicine approaches by using patient-specific cells to create disease models or test drugs. This allows for more accurate predictions of drug efficacy and toxicity, leading to safer and more efficient treatments.

In conclusion, ex vivo engineering is a cutting-edge field within tissue engineering that offers tremendous potential for revolutionizing regenerative medicine. By harnessing the principles of materials science and engineering, researchers are creating innovative biomaterials that can support cell growth, tissue regeneration, and organ transplantation. The applications of ex vivo engineering are far-reaching, spanning from repairing damaged tissues to advancing personalized medicine. As this field continues to advance, we can look forward to a future where ex vivo engineering plays a pivotal role in building a better tomorrow for medical science and patient care.

Chapter 6: Applications of Tissue Engineering

Skin Tissue Engineering

Skin tissue engineering is a revolutionary field that aims to address the challenges associated with skin regeneration and repair. The human skin is an essential organ that serves as a protective barrier against external threats, such as pathogens and physical injuries. However, it is also prone to damage from burns, chronic wounds, and congenital defects. Traditional treatment methods, such as skin grafts, have limitations and may result in scarring, infection, and a lack of functional and aesthetic outcomes. This is where skin tissue engineering provides a promising solution.

Skin tissue engineering involves the development and fabrication of biomaterials and scaffolds that can mimic the structure and function of native skin. These biomaterials are specifically designed to support cell adhesion, proliferation, and differentiation, enabling the growth of new skin tissue. The materials used in this process must be biocompatible, non-toxic, and possess suitable mechanical properties.

Materials science and engineering play a crucial role in the success of skin tissue engineering. Researchers in this field are constantly exploring new materials and fabrication techniques to improve the outcomes of skin regeneration. For instance, biodegradable polymers, such as poly(lactic-co-glycolic acid) (PLGA) and polycaprolactone (PCL), have been extensively studied for their ability to provide temporary scaffolds that degrade over time, allowing for the integration of new tissue.

In addition to biomaterials, the use of stem cells and growth factors is another important aspect of skin tissue engineering. Stem cells have the potential to differentiate into various cell types, including skin cells, and can be utilized to enhance the regeneration process. Growth factors, such as transforming growth factor-beta (TGF-β) and platelet-derived growth factor (PDGF), can stimulate cell migration, proliferation, and extracellular matrix production, facilitating the formation of new skin tissue.

Moreover, advanced techniques like 3D printing have revolutionized the field of skin tissue engineering. By utilizing bioprinting technology, researchers can precisely deposit cells and biomaterials layer by layer, creating complex structures that closely resemble native skin. This technique allows for the customization of scaffolds according to the patient's specific needs, enhancing the efficacy and efficiency of skin regeneration therapies.

In conclusion, skin tissue engineering holds immense potential for the future of regenerative medicine. With the continuous advancements in materials science and engineering, researchers are working towards building a better tomorrow where functional and aesthetically pleasing skin can be regenerated. This interdisciplinary field has the potential to revolutionize the treatment of burns, chronic wounds, and various skin defects, ultimately improving the quality of life for countless individuals worldwide.

Burns and Wound Healing

In the quest to build a better tomorrow, one cannot overlook the importance of advancements in the field of materials science and engineering, particularly when it comes to burns and wound healing. Burns are one of the most common and painful injuries, affecting people of all ages and backgrounds. Wound healing, on the other hand, is a complex biological process that involves the regeneration of damaged tissue. With the help of innovative materials, scientists and engineers are revolutionizing the way we treat burns and enhance wound healing.

Traditional methods of burn treatment have often relied on the use of skin grafts, which involve transplanting healthy skin from one area of the body to another. While this approach has proven effective, it is limited by the availability of donor sites and the risk of complications. However, materials science and engineering have introduced novel alternatives that can revolutionize burn treatment.

One such innovation is the development of biomaterials that promote skin regeneration. These materials can be designed to mimic the natural extracellular matrix, providing a scaffold for the growth of new skin cells. By combining synthetic polymers with natural components, these biomaterials offer a biocompatible and biodegradable solution for burn wound healing. Furthermore, the integration of growth factors and drug delivery systems within these materials can enhance the healing process and prevent infection.

Additionally, the use of nanomaterials has opened up new possibilities in the field of burns and wound healing. Nanofibers, for instance, can be electrospun to create a scaffold with a high surface area-to-volume ratio, facilitating cell adhesion and proliferation. Nanoparticles, on the other hand, can be loaded with therapeutics and targeted to the site of injury, offering a localized and controlled release of drugs. These nanomaterials hold immense potential for the development of advanced dressings and bandages that can accelerate wound healing and minimize scarring.

By harnessing the power of materials science and engineering, researchers are paving the way for a future where burns and wound healing can be treated more effectively and efficiently. These advancements not only promise relief for patients but also offer opportunities for more sustainable and cost-effective solutions. As we continue to explore and innovate in this field, the possibilities for building a better tomorrow become increasingly within reach.

Skin Grafts

Skin grafts have revolutionized the field of tissue engineering, providing hope and healing for individuals suffering from severe injuries or burns. This subchapter explores the use of skin grafts in regenerative medicine and the materials science behind their success.

Skin grafts involve the transplantation of skin from one area of the body, known as the donor site, to another area that has been damaged or lost due to injury or disease. They play a crucial role in restoring the function and appearance of the skin, promoting wound healing, and preventing infection.

Materials science and engineering have played a significant role in the development of skin grafts. Researchers have explored various biomaterials to create scaffolds that mimic the natural structure and function of human skin. These scaffolds provide a framework for the growth of new cells, blood vessels, and other components necessary for tissue regeneration.

One commonly used material for skin grafts is collagen, a biocompatible protein that forms the building blocks of the extracellular matrix in our skin. Collagen-based scaffolds can be engineered to have specific properties, such as pore size and mechanical strength, to support cell attachment and proliferation. Additionally, synthetic polymers like polyglycolic acid (PGA) and polylactic acid (PLA) have been utilized to create scaffolds with tailored properties.

In recent years, advances in stem cell research have further enhanced the potential of skin grafts. Researchers have successfully used induced pluripotent stem cells (iPSCs) to generate functional skin tissue. These iPSCs can be derived from a patient's own cells, reducing the risk of rejection and increasing the success rate of grafts.

Moreover, the development of innovative techniques, such as 3D printing, has allowed for the fabrication of complex skin grafts with precise structures and patient-specific designs. This technology enables the creation of multilayered grafts that closely resemble natural skin, enhancing their regenerative capabilities.

In conclusion, skin grafts have become a vital tool in tissue engineering, offering hope to patients with severe skin injuries or burns. The field of materials science and engineering has played a crucial role in the development of effective and innovative grafts. By utilizing biomaterials, stem cells, and advanced manufacturing techniques, researchers continue to push the boundaries of what is possible, building a better tomorrow for patients in need of skin regeneration.

Artificial Skin Substitutes

In the field of tissue engineering, one of the most significant advancements has been the development of artificial skin substitutes. These substitutes are designed to mimic the structure and function of natural skin, providing a viable solution for patients with severe burns, chronic wounds, or other skin-related injuries. This subchapter will explore the materials used in artificial skin substitutes and their applications, highlighting the incredible potential they hold in the field of medicine.

Materials Science and Engineering have played a crucial role in the development of artificial skin substitutes. Researchers have focused on selecting materials that possess the necessary mechanical, biological, and physiological properties to closely resemble natural skin. Synthetic polymers, such as poly(lactic-co-glycolic acid) (PLGA) and polycaprolactone (PCL), have been extensively used due to their biocompatibility and tunable degradation rates. These materials provide a structural scaffold that allows cells to adhere and proliferate, promoting tissue regeneration.

In addition to synthetic polymers, natural biomaterials have also been explored as potential components of artificial skin substitutes. Collagen, the most abundant protein in the human body, has shown great promise in enhancing cell attachment and promoting wound healing. Other natural materials, like chitosan and hyaluronic acid, have also demonstrated their ability to support cell growth and improve tissue integration.

The fabrication techniques used to create artificial skin substitutes are crucial in determining their properties and functionality. Techniques such as electrospinning, 3D bioprinting, and spray deposition have been employed to create highly porous scaffolds that closely resemble the architecture of natural skin. These scaffolds provide a framework for cells to populate and differentiate, facilitating the regeneration of functional skin tissue.

The applications of artificial skin substitutes are vast and diverse. They have proven to be particularly useful in the treatment of burn injuries, where large areas of damaged skin need to be replaced. These substitutes can also be used in chronic wound management, providing a supportive environment for wound healing and reducing the risk of infection. Moreover, artificial skin substitutes hold great potential in the field of cosmetic and reconstructive surgery, allowing for more natural and seamless results.

In conclusion, the development of artificial skin substitutes is a significant breakthrough in the field of tissue engineering. Through the use of innovative materials and fabrication techniques, researchers have been able to create substitutes that closely resemble natural skin, providing hope for patients with severe skin injuries. The advancements made in this area have the potential to revolutionize medical treatments and improve the quality of life for millions of people worldwide.

Bone Tissue Engineering

Bone tissue engineering is a rapidly advancing field within the broader discipline of tissue engineering, with the goal of developing new and improved methods for repairing and regenerating damaged or lost bone tissue. This subchapter explores the various materials and techniques used in bone tissue engineering, highlighting their potential to revolutionize the field and improve patient outcomes.

Bone is a complex and dynamic tissue that provides structural support for the body, protects vital organs, and facilitates movement. However, it is susceptible to damage and degeneration due to trauma, disease, and aging. Traditional approaches to bone repair, such as bone grafts or metal implants, have limitations and often result in suboptimal outcomes. Bone tissue engineering offers a promising alternative by combining principles of materials science and engineering with the regenerative capacity of the body.

One of the key challenges in bone tissue engineering is finding suitable materials that can mimic the properties of natural bone and provide a scaffold for new bone growth. Biocompatible materials, such as polymers, ceramics, and composites, are extensively researched for their ability to support cell attachment, proliferation, and differentiation. These materials can be fabricated into three-dimensional scaffolds with controlled porosity and mechanical properties, allowing cells to infiltrate and deposit new bone tissue.

In addition to materials, the field of bone tissue engineering also explores various techniques to enhance bone regeneration. These include the use of growth factors, such as bone morphogenetic proteins (BMPs), which can stimulate the differentiation of mesenchymal stem cells into bone-forming cells. Scaffold functionalization with bioactive molecules and surface modification techniques can further enhance cell-material interactions and promote bone tissue formation.

Furthermore, advancements in additive manufacturing, commonly known as 3D printing, have revolutionized bone tissue engineering. This technology allows for the precise fabrication of patient-specific scaffolds with complex geometries, enabling better integration with surrounding tissues and improved functional outcomes.

Bone tissue engineering holds tremendous potential in the field of regenerative medicine, offering new hope for patients with bone defects or skeletal disorders. By combining materials science and engineering principles, researchers are developing innovative solutions to overcome the limitations of traditional bone repair methods. The ongoing advancements in this field are paving the way for a future where damaged bone tissue can be regenerated, leading to improved quality of life and better patient outcomes.

In conclusion, bone tissue engineering is a rapidly evolving field that combines materials science and engineering principles to develop innovative solutions for bone repair and regeneration. Through the use of biocompatible materials, growth factors, and advanced fabrication techniques, researchers are working towards building a better tomorrow where damaged bone tissue can be fully restored, thereby improving the lives of countless individuals.

Bone Defect Repair

Bone defects can occur due to a variety of reasons such as trauma, infection, tumors, or congenital disorders. These defects can significantly impact an individual's quality of life, resulting in pain, limited mobility, and compromised skeletal structure. However, with advancements in materials science and engineering, there is hope for a better tomorrow in the field of bone defect repair.

One of the key approaches for bone defect repair is the use of tissue engineering. Tissue engineering involves the design and fabrication of biomaterials that can provide a scaffold for cells to grow and regenerate bone tissue. These biomaterials can be synthetic or natural, and they play a crucial role in guiding the repair process.

In recent years, a wide range of materials have been explored for bone defect repair. Synthetic materials such as bioceramics, polymers, and metals have shown promising results. Bioceramics, like hydroxyapatite and tricalcium phosphate, have excellent biocompatibility and can mimic the mineral composition of natural bone. Polymers, such as poly(lactic-co-glycolic acid) and poly(caprolactone), offer versatility in terms of mechanical properties and degradation rates. Metals like titanium and stainless steel are commonly used for load-bearing applications due to their high strength and durability.

Natural materials, including collagen, chitosan, and demineralized bone matrix, have also been utilized for bone defect repair. These materials possess inherent biological properties that can promote cell attachment, proliferation, and differentiation. Collagen, in particular, is a widely used natural material due to its biocompatibility and ability to support cell growth.

In addition to biomaterials, growth factors and stem cells are key players in bone defect repair. Growth factors, such as bone morphogenetic proteins, can stimulate the differentiation of stem cells into bone-forming cells. Stem cells, including mesenchymal stem cells and induced pluripotent stem cells, have the potential to differentiate into various cell types, including osteoblasts, which are responsible for bone formation.

Furthermore, advancements in additive manufacturing technologies, such as 3D printing, have revolutionized the field of bone defect repair. 3D printing allows for the fabrication of patient-specific scaffolds with complex geometries that can precisely fit the defect site. This personalized approach enhances the integration of the scaffold with the surrounding bone tissue, leading to improved healing outcomes.

In conclusion, the field of bone defect repair has witnessed significant advancements in materials science and engineering. The use of biomaterials, growth factors, stem cells, and additive manufacturing technologies has opened up new possibilities for effective bone regeneration. With ongoing research and innovation, the future of bone defect repair looks promising, offering hope for a better tomorrow for individuals suffering from bone defects.

Bone Grafts and Substitutes

Bone grafts and substitutes play a crucial role in the field of tissue engineering, providing a solution to the challenges faced in bone repair and regeneration. These materials are designed to mimic the natural bone structure and enhance the body's ability to heal itself, making them essential in various medical procedures. This subchapter will delve into the world of bone grafts and substitutes, exploring their composition, types, and applications.

Bone grafts are materials used to replace or repair damaged or missing bone in the body. They are often derived from the patient's own bone (autografts), donor bone (allografts), or synthetic materials (alloplasts). Autografts have been the gold standard for bone grafting due to their excellent biocompatibility and osteogenic properties. However, harvesting autografts requires an additional surgical site, leading to increased pain and morbidity. Allografts offer an alternative, but the risk of disease transmission and immunological rejection remains a concern. Alloplasts, on the other hand, are synthetic materials that eliminate these risks but lack the biological properties necessary for optimal bone regeneration.

To address the limitations of traditional bone grafts, researchers have developed various substitutes that combine the benefits of autografts and alloplasts. These substitutes are typically composed of biocompatible materials, such as ceramics, polymers, or composite materials. Ceramics, including hydroxyapatite and calcium phosphate, closely resemble the mineral phase of bone, providing a scaffold for new bone formation. Polymers, such as biodegradable polymers, offer flexibility and mechanical strength while degrading over time, allowing for new bone growth. Composite materials combine the advantages of both ceramics and polymers, promoting cell adhesion and proliferation.

The applications of bone grafts and substitutes are vast, ranging from dental implants and spinal fusions to complex reconstructive surgeries. These materials can bridge bone defects, promote bone fusion, and enhance bone regeneration. Additionally, they can be used as carriers for growth factors, drugs, or cells, further enhancing their therapeutic potential. The field of bone tissue engineering continues to evolve, with ongoing research focused on improving the mechanical properties, bioactivity, and biodegradability of bone grafts and substitutes.

In summary, bone grafts and substitutes are vital tools in the field of tissue engineering, providing solutions to bone repair and regeneration. With their diverse composition and applications, these materials have the potential to revolutionize the way we treat bone-related injuries and diseases. As materials scientists and engineers continue to innovate and refine these technologies, the future of bone grafts and substitutes holds great promise for a better tomorrow.

Osteochondral Tissue Engineering

In recent years, tissue engineering has emerged as a promising field in the quest to regenerate damaged or diseased tissues. One area of focus within this field is osteochondral tissue engineering, which aims to repair or replace damaged bone and cartilage. This subchapter will delve into the fascinating world of osteochondral tissue engineering, exploring the materials and techniques used to build a better tomorrow for patients suffering from osteochondral defects.

Osteochondral defects, characterized by the loss or damage of both bone and cartilage, pose a significant challenge for traditional treatment approaches. Conventional therapies often fail to fully restore the native tissue structure and function, leading to pain, limited mobility, and reduced quality of life for patients. However, tissue engineering offers a promising solution by combining biomaterials, cells, and growth factors to develop functional and biocompatible constructs that can regenerate damaged tissue.

Materials science and engineering play a crucial role in osteochondral tissue engineering. A variety of materials, such as natural polymers, synthetic polymers, ceramics, and composites, have been explored for their ability to mimic the native extracellular matrix (ECM) and provide mechanical support to the regenerating tissue. These materials must possess the appropriate mechanical properties, biocompatibility, and degradation rates to support cell attachment, proliferation, and differentiation.

In addition to biomaterials, the use of stem cells is a key component in osteochondral tissue engineering. Mesenchymal stem cells (MSCs) have shown great potential in differentiating into bone and cartilage cells, making them an ideal candidate for regenerating osteochondral defects. Scaffold-based approaches, where MSCs are seeded onto biomaterial scaffolds, provide a suitable microenvironment for cell growth and tissue formation.

Furthermore, advances in bioreactor technology have enabled the development of dynamic culture systems that enhance cell proliferation, differentiation, and tissue formation. Bioreactors can provide mechanical stimulation, nutrient supply, and waste removal, mimicking the physiological conditions necessary for tissue development. These systems have shown promising results in promoting the formation of functional osteochondral tissue constructs.

In conclusion, osteochondral tissue engineering holds great promise for the regeneration of damaged bone and cartilage. Through the integration of materials science and engineering, researchers are developing innovative approaches to overcome the limitations of traditional treatments. By combining biomaterials, stem cells, and bioreactor technology, osteochondral tissue engineering aims to restore the structure and function of damaged tissues, improving the lives of patients suffering from osteochondral defects. The ongoing advancements in this field bring hope for a future where regenerative medicine becomes a reality for everyone.

Cartilage Tissue Engineering

In recent years, the field of tissue engineering has emerged as a promising approach to address the limitations of conventional treatments for cartilage defects and injuries. Cartilage tissue engineering combines principles from materials science and engineering to develop innovative strategies for repairing or regenerating damaged cartilage.

Cartilage is a specialized connective tissue found in various parts of the body, including the joints, ears, and nose. It plays a crucial role in providing cushioning and support to the joints, facilitating smooth movement, and maintaining the structural integrity of the body. However, cartilage has limited self-healing capacity, making it prone to degeneration and damage caused by aging, trauma, or certain diseases such as osteoarthritis.

Materials science and engineering have paved the way for the development of biomaterials that can mimic the properties of native cartilage and promote tissue regeneration. These biomaterials act as scaffolds that provide structural support and create a favorable environment for cells to grow and differentiate into functional cartilage tissue.

One of the key challenges in cartilage tissue engineering is finding suitable biomaterials that possess the necessary mechanical and biological properties to support cartilage regeneration. Researchers have explored a wide range of materials, including natural polymers such as collagen and chitosan, as well as synthetic polymers like poly(lactic-co-glycolic acid) (PLGA) and poly(ethylene glycol) (PEG).

These materials can be engineered to have specific characteristics, such as porosity and mechanical strength, to meet the requirements of cartilage tissue engineering.

In addition to biomaterials, cells play a critical role in cartilage tissue engineering. Various cell sources, including chondrocytes (cartilage cells) and mesenchymal stem cells (MSCs), have been investigated for their potential to regenerate cartilage. These cells can be seeded onto the biomaterial scaffolds and cultured in the laboratory to promote the formation of cartilage tissue. Moreover, researchers are exploring the use of growth factors and bioactive molecules to enhance cell survival, proliferation, and differentiation.

Cartilage tissue engineering holds great promise for improving the treatment outcomes of cartilage defects and injuries. By harnessing the principles of materials science and engineering, researchers are developing innovative strategies to regenerate functional cartilage tissue and restore joint function. Continued advancements in this field will not only benefit patients suffering from cartilage-related conditions but also contribute to the broader field of tissue engineering, paving the way for a better tomorrow in healthcare.

Articular Cartilage Repair

Articular cartilage is a crucial component of our joints, providing a smooth, low-friction surface that allows for pain-free movement. However, it is prone to injury and degeneration, leading to conditions such as osteoarthritis. Fortunately, advancements in materials science and engineering have paved the way for innovative approaches to repair and regenerate articular cartilage, offering hope for a better tomorrow.

Articular cartilage has a limited capacity for self-repair due to its avascular nature and low cellularity. Traditional treatments such as pain management and joint replacement have limitations in terms of long-term efficacy and patient satisfaction. Therefore, tissue engineering strategies have emerged as a promising solution to address this unmet clinical need.

One approach to articular cartilage repair involves the use of biomaterials, which can provide structural support and promote the growth of new cartilage tissue. Biocompatible scaffolds made from natural or synthetic materials serve as templates for cell attachment and proliferation. These scaffolds can be seeded with chondrocytes, the cells responsible for cartilage production, or stem cells capable of differentiating into chondrocytes. In addition, bioactive molecules such as growth factors can be incorporated into the scaffolds to enhance tissue regeneration.

Another exciting avenue for articular cartilage repair is the development of 3D printing technologies. By using computer-aided design (CAD) models, customized scaffolds with precise dimensions and architecture can be fabricated. This allows for the creation of patient-specific implants that closely mimic the native cartilage structure, promoting integration and enhancing functional outcomes.

Furthermore, ongoing research focuses on the development of smart materials that respond to mechanical stimuli. These materials can mimic the dynamic nature of articular cartilage, adapting to changes in joint loading and providing optimal mechanical properties. By harnessing the power of materials science and engineering, scientists are striving to create biomimetic materials that can not only repair damaged cartilage but also restore its native functionality.

In conclusion, articular cartilage repair is an exciting field that holds great potential for improving the lives of millions suffering from joint pain and disability. Through the integration of materials science and engineering principles, researchers aim to develop innovative strategies to repair and regenerate articular cartilage. These advancements in the field of tissue engineering offer hope for a future where patients can regain pain-free movement and enjoy a better quality of life.

Meniscus Repair

The meniscus is a crucial part of the knee joint that acts as a shock absorber and provides stability during movement. However, it is prone to injuries, especially in physically active individuals. Meniscus tears are a common occurrence and can significantly impact one's quality of life. In recent years, materials science and engineering have made remarkable advancements in the field of meniscus repair, leading to the development of innovative techniques and materials that help restore the function and integrity of the meniscus.

This subchapter aims to provide a comprehensive overview of meniscus repair techniques and the materials used in the process. It is intended for a diverse audience, including medical professionals, researchers, and individuals interested in the field of materials science and engineering.

The subchapter begins by exploring the different types of meniscus tears and their classification based on severity and location. It delves into the challenges associated with meniscus repair, such as the limited blood supply and the complex anatomy of the knee joint. The subchapter then introduces the concept of tissue engineering and its application in meniscus repair.

Materials science and engineering play a crucial role in developing scaffolds and biomaterials that promote meniscus regeneration. The subchapter discusses various materials used in meniscus repair, including natural and synthetic polymers, hydrogels, and biocompatible metals. It highlights their properties, advantages, and limitations, providing readers with an understanding of the selection criteria for different materials in meniscus repair.

Furthermore, the subchapter explores emerging techniques such as 3D printing and nanotechnology in meniscus repair. It discusses their potential in fabricating patient-specific scaffolds and enhancing the healing process. Additionally, it covers the importance of biomechanical considerations in meniscus repair, emphasizing the need for materials that mimic the mechanical properties of the native meniscus.

The subchapter also addresses the challenges and future directions in meniscus repair. It discusses the need for long-term studies to evaluate the efficacy and safety of new materials and techniques. It also highlights the importance of multidisciplinary collaborations between materials scientists, engineers, and medical professionals to develop better solutions for meniscus repair.

In conclusion, this subchapter provides a comprehensive overview of meniscus repair, focusing on the materials science and engineering aspects. It aims to educate a diverse audience about the current state of meniscus repair techniques and the potential for future advancements. By understanding the materials and techniques involved in meniscus repair, we can work towards building a better tomorrow for individuals suffering from meniscus injuries.

Organ and Vascular Tissue Engineering

In recent years, the field of tissue engineering has emerged as a promising solution to the growing demand for organ and vascular transplantation. This subchapter explores the fascinating realm of organ and vascular tissue engineering, showcasing how materials science and engineering have played a pivotal role in advancing this cutting-edge field.

Organ transplantation has long been the gold standard for treating end-stage organ failure. However, the scarcity of donor organs and the risk of rejection have limited its effectiveness. Tissue engineering offers a revolutionary alternative by creating functional organs in the laboratory, using a combination of cells, biomaterials, and bioactive molecules.

One of the key challenges in organ engineering is recreating the complex architecture and functionality of natural organs. Materials science and engineering have provided innovative solutions by developing 3D scaffolds that mimic the extracellular matrix, the natural environment where cells reside. These scaffolds act as a framework for cell growth, allowing them to organize, differentiate, and develop into specific organ tissues.

The choice of materials used in organ engineering is crucial. Biocompatible polymers, such as hydrogels, play a vital role in providing mechanical support while allowing nutrient and oxygen diffusion to the cells. Additionally, bioactive molecules, such as growth factors, can be incorporated into the scaffolds to guide cell behavior and promote tissue regeneration.

The vascular system plays a vital role in delivering oxygen and nutrients to organs. Vascular tissue engineering aims to create functional blood vessels that can integrate with the host's circulatory system. Materials science and engineering have made significant advancements in this area by developing biomaterials that can support the growth of endothelial cells, the building blocks of blood vessels. These biomaterials can be designed to have specific mechanical properties, surface topographies, and biochemical cues to promote vasculogenesis and angiogenesis.

Moreover, advances in bioprinting technology have allowed researchers to fabricate complex vascular networks within engineered organs. This breakthrough has brought us closer to the goal of creating fully functional organs for transplantation.

Organ and vascular tissue engineering hold tremendous promise for the future of medicine. By harnessing the power of materials science and engineering, researchers are working towards building a better tomorrow where the shortage of donor organs is alleviated, and patients can receive life-saving treatments without the risk of rejection.

Liver Tissue Engineering

Liver tissue engineering is an exciting and rapidly expanding field that holds great promise for the future of medicine. The liver is a vital organ responsible for a wide range of functions, including detoxification, metabolism, and the production of essential proteins. Unfortunately, liver diseases such as cirrhosis and liver failure are common and pose significant challenges for patients and healthcare professionals alike.

Traditional treatment methods for liver diseases, such as liver transplantation, are often limited by the shortage of donor organs and the risk of rejection. Liver tissue engineering offers a potential solution to these problems by creating functional liver tissue in the laboratory.

Materials science and engineering play a crucial role in liver tissue engineering, as they provide the tools and techniques necessary to create liver-like structures that closely mimic the native tissue. The use of biocompatible and biodegradable materials, such as hydrogels and scaffolds, allows for the growth and organization of liver cells in a three-dimensional environment. These materials provide the necessary support and cues for the cells to differentiate and function properly.

In addition to materials, the field of liver tissue engineering also relies on advances in cell biology and tissue culture techniques. Liver cells, or hepatocytes, can be obtained from various sources, including donated livers, stem cells, or even reprogrammed skin cells. These cells can then be cultured and expanded in the laboratory before being seeded onto the scaffolds or hydrogels. By providing the appropriate growth factors and nutrients, researchers can encourage the cells to grow and develop into functional liver tissue.

One of the main challenges in liver tissue engineering is creating a vascular network that can supply the growing tissue with nutrients and oxygen. Without a functional blood supply, the tissue would quickly die. Researchers are exploring various strategies to address this issue, including the use of biofabrication techniques to create blood vessel-like structures within the engineered tissue.

The ultimate goal of liver tissue engineering is to develop functional liver tissue that can be used for transplantation or as a model for drug testing and disease research. While there is still much work to be done, the field holds great promise for improving the lives of patients with liver diseases and advancing our understanding of liver biology. Through the collaboration of materials science and engineering, we can build a better tomorrow for liver tissue engineering and the field of regenerative medicine as a whole.

Heart Tissue Engineering

In recent years, the field of tissue engineering has emerged as a promising approach to tackle the growing need for viable organ replacements. One particular area of focus within tissue engineering is heart tissue engineering, which aims to create functional cardiac tissue for transplantation or as a model for drug testing and disease research. This subchapter explores the principles and advancements in heart tissue engineering, highlighting the crucial role of materials science and engineering in this field.

The heart is a remarkable organ with complex structures and functions, making it challenging to replicate artificially. However, with advancements in biomaterials and cell culture techniques, scientists have made significant progress in creating engineered heart tissues that closely resemble native heart tissue. The key to successful heart tissue engineering lies in the selection of appropriate materials and their precise integration with cells.

Materials science and engineering play a vital role in heart tissue engineering by providing scaffolds and biomaterials that mimic the native extracellular matrix (ECM) of the heart. The ECM provides structural support and biochemical cues necessary for cell adhesion, proliferation, and differentiation. Researchers have developed various biomaterials, including natural polymers like collagen and synthetic polymers such as polyglycolic acid (PGA) and polylactic acid (PLA). These materials can be processed into porous scaffolds with specific mechanical and biochemical properties to guide cell behavior and tissue growth.

In addition to scaffolds, materials are also utilized to deliver cells and bioactive molecules to the engineered heart tissue. Cell sources for heart tissue engineering include embryonic stem cells, induced pluripotent stem cells, and adult cardiac progenitor cells. These cells are often combined with growth factors and cytokines to promote cell survival, proliferation, and differentiation. Materials such as hydrogels, microspheres, and nanoparticles are used as carriers for controlled release of these bioactive molecules.

Furthermore, materials science plays a crucial role in developing techniques for monitoring and assessing the functionality of engineered heart tissues. Advanced imaging techniques, such as MRI and ultrasound, provide valuable information about tissue morphology and function. Additionally, materials with integrated sensors and microelectrodes enable real-time monitoring of electrical signals and contractile properties of the engineered tissues.

Heart tissue engineering holds immense potential in revolutionizing the treatment of cardiovascular diseases by providing personalized and regenerative therapies. However, several challenges remain, including the need for improved vascularization and electrical integration of the engineered tissues. Continued research in materials science and engineering will be instrumental in overcoming these obstacles and building a better tomorrow for patients suffering from heart diseases.

This subchapter serves as a comprehensive introduction to heart tissue engineering, emphasizing the critical role of materials science and engineering in advancing this field. It aims to provide a broad understanding of the principles and challenges involved in creating functional cardiac tissue, making it accessible to a wide audience, including researchers, students, and healthcare professionals interested in the field of tissue engineering.

Blood Vessel Engineering

In the field of tissue engineering, one of the most critical challenges is the creation and regeneration of functional blood vessels. Blood vessels play a vital role in delivering oxygen and nutrients to tissues, as well as removing waste products. Without a well-functioning vascular system, engineered tissues would not survive or thrive. That is why blood vessel engineering has emerged as a cutting-edge field in materials science and engineering.

Traditionally, tissue engineering strategies have focused on creating scaffolds that mimic the extracellular matrix (ECM), the natural environment in which cells reside. However, the design and fabrication of blood vessels bring additional complexities due to their unique structure and function. Blood vessels consist of a lining of endothelial cells, surrounded by smooth muscle cells, and are supported by a network of collagen and elastin fibers. Thus, the development of biomaterials that can replicate these intricate characteristics is crucial.

Researchers have made significant progress in this field by exploring various materials and fabrication techniques. One approach involves using biodegradable polymers as scaffolds. These polymers can be processed into porous structures that allow cell infiltration and promote tissue integration. Additionally, they can be loaded with growth factors or drugs to enhance the development and functionality of blood vessels.

Another promising strategy is the use of bioactive materials that can stimulate the growth and differentiation of endothelial and smooth muscle cells. These materials can be functionalized with bioactive molecules, such as peptides or growth factors, which can interact with cell receptors and trigger specific cellular responses. By mimicking the natural signaling mechanisms, these materials can guide the formation of blood vessels and promote their maturation.

Furthermore, advanced fabrication techniques, such as 3D printing and electrospinning, have been employed to create complex and precise blood vessel structures. These techniques allow the fabrication of patient-specific blood vessels, which can greatly enhance the success of tissue engineering therapies. Additionally, the incorporation of microchannels within the scaffolds can mimic the hierarchical structure of native blood vessels, further improving their functionality.

In conclusion, blood vessel engineering is a rapidly evolving field within materials science and engineering that aims to develop functional and biomimetic blood vessels for tissue engineering applications. Through the use of biodegradable polymers, bioactive materials, and advanced fabrication techniques, researchers are making tremendous strides in creating blood vessel scaffolds that can support the growth and regeneration of tissues. The advancements in this field hold great promise for the development of more effective tissue engineering therapies, ultimately leading to a better tomorrow for patients in need of regenerative treatments.

Chapter 7: Regulatory and Ethical Considerations in Tissue Engineering

Regulatory Frameworks and Approval Process

In the field of tissue engineering, the development and utilization of new materials play a vital role in creating innovative solutions for regenerative medicine. However, ensuring the safety and efficacy of these materials before they can be used in clinical settings is of utmost importance. This subchapter aims to provide an overview of the regulatory frameworks and approval processes involved in bringing tissue engineering materials from the laboratory to the bedside.

Materials science and engineering researchers are constantly exploring new materials and fabrication techniques that hold promise for tissue engineering applications. These materials may range from biocompatible polymers and ceramics to natural biomaterials and composite scaffolds. However, before these materials can be utilized for therapeutic purposes, they must undergo stringent evaluations and approval processes to ensure their safety and efficacy.

Regulatory agencies, such as the Food and Drug Administration (FDA) in the United States, have established guidelines and regulations to evaluate the safety and effectiveness of tissue engineering materials. These regulations are designed to protect patients from potential risks associated with new materials and therapies, while also fostering innovation in the field.

The approval process for tissue engineering materials typically involves several stages, starting with preclinical testing in laboratory settings. This includes in vitro experiments to assess the biocompatibility and functionality of the materials, as well as animal studies to evaluate their performance in living systems. The results from these studies are then submitted to regulatory agencies for review.

If the preclinical data show promising results, the material can proceed to clinical trials, which involve testing on human subjects. Clinical trials are conducted in multiple phases, with each phase focusing on different aspects such as safety, dosage optimization, and efficacy. The data obtained from these trials are carefully analyzed and presented to regulatory bodies to support the approval process.

Once a tissue engineering material successfully completes the approval process, it can be utilized in clinical practice. However, post-market surveillance is essential to monitor the long-term safety and effectiveness of these materials. This continuous evaluation allows regulatory agencies to update guidelines and regulations if necessary, ensuring that the field of tissue engineering continues to evolve and improve.

In conclusion, the regulatory frameworks and approval process for tissue engineering materials are critical in ensuring their safety and efficacy. Materials scientists and engineers play a crucial role in developing innovative materials, but their work must be guided by regulatory guidelines and evaluated through rigorous testing. By adhering to these processes, we can ensure that tissue engineering continues to build a better tomorrow for patients in need of regenerative medicine solutions.

Ethical Considerations in Tissue Engineering Research

Tissue engineering has emerged as a promising field that holds the potential to revolutionize healthcare by creating functional and viable tissues and organs. However, as with any scientific advancement, there are ethical considerations that need to be addressed to ensure responsible and sustainable progress in tissue engineering research. This subchapter explores the ethical dimensions of tissue engineering and the critical issues that researchers and stakeholders must grapple with.

One of the foremost ethical considerations in tissue engineering research is informed consent. The use of human tissues and cells in research should be conducted with the explicit consent of donors or their legally authorized representatives. Researchers must ensure that potential donors fully understand the purpose, risks, and potential benefits of their contributions. Additionally, privacy and confidentiality of donors' personal information and genetic data must be protected to maintain their dignity and autonomy.

Another ethical concern revolves around the sourcing of materials for tissue engineering. The use of animal tissues, embryonic stem cells, or other biological materials raises questions about animal welfare and the moral status of embryos. Researchers should strive to minimize the use of animals in their experiments and explore alternative sources of cells, such as induced pluripotent stem cells, which do not involve the destruction of embryos.

Equitable access to tissue engineering therapies is another pressing ethical issue. As this field progresses, it is crucial to ensure that novel treatments are affordable and accessible to all members of society, regardless of their socioeconomic status or geographic location. Efforts should be made to avoid exacerbating existing health disparities and to prioritize the public interest over commercial interests.

Furthermore, the potential for unintended consequences and long-term effects of tissue engineering should not be overlooked. Researchers must conduct thorough risk assessments and carefully evaluate the potential benefits and harms of their interventions. Transparent communication with the public about the uncertainty and limitations surrounding tissue engineering is essential to foster trust and manage expectations.

Lastly, the intellectual property landscape in tissue engineering research raises ethical concerns. Patents and exclusive licensing agreements can hinder collaboration, restrict access to knowledge, and impede further scientific advancements. Researchers should strive to strike a balance between protecting intellectual property rights and promoting the open exchange of information for the benefit of society as a whole.

In conclusion, tissue engineering research holds great promise for improving human health and well-being. However, it is essential to approach this field with a strong ethical framework. Informed consent, responsible material sourcing, equitable access, risk assessment, transparent communication, and collaborative research practices are all crucial aspects of ethical tissue engineering. By addressing these ethical considerations, we can ensure that tissue engineering research is conducted in a socially responsible manner, leading to a better tomorrow for all.

Future Challenges and Directions in Tissue Engineering

As the field of tissue engineering continues to advance, the future holds both exciting opportunities and significant challenges. This chapter explores the potential directions and hurdles that lie ahead, offering a glimpse into what the future of tissue engineering may look like.

One of the key challenges in tissue engineering is the development of biomaterials that can closely mimic the complex structure and properties of native tissues. While significant progress has been made in this area, there is still much work to be done. Researchers are exploring novel materials and fabrication techniques to create scaffolds that can guide cell growth and differentiation in a more precise manner. The goal is to create biomaterials that not only provide mechanical support but also promote cellular activities, such as signaling and communication, to better mimic the natural extracellular matrix.

Another critical challenge is vascularization, or the formation of blood vessels within engineered tissues. Without a proper blood supply, larger and more complex tissues cannot survive. Researchers are exploring various strategies, including the use of microfluidic systems and 3D bioprinting, to create functional blood vessel networks within engineered tissues. These advancements will be crucial for the successful transplantation of artificial organs and the treatment of various diseases.

In addition to technical challenges, ethical considerations are also emerging in tissue engineering. The ability to create personalized tissues and organs raises questions about ownership, consent, and the potential commodification of human body parts. It is essential for scientists, policymakers, and society as a whole to engage in discussions and establish ethical guidelines to ensure the responsible development and use of tissue engineering technologies.

Looking ahead, tissue engineering holds great promise for regenerative medicine, disease modeling, and drug testing. The ability to engineer tissues that closely resemble human organs will revolutionize the field of drug discovery, as it will enable more accurate and efficient screening of potential therapeutics. Furthermore, tissue engineering has the potential to provide solutions for organ transplantation, alleviating the shortage of donor organs and reducing the risk of rejection.

In conclusion, the future of tissue engineering is full of possibilities and challenges. The development of biomaterials that closely mimic native tissues, the vascularization of engineered tissues, and the ethical considerations associated with tissue engineering are some of the key areas that need further exploration. However, with continued advancements in materials science and engineering, tissue engineering holds the promise of building a better tomorrow for regenerative medicine and beyond.

Chapter 8: Conclusion and Future Outlook

Summary of Key Findings

As we delve into the fascinating world of tissue engineering, we uncover groundbreaking research and discoveries that have the potential to revolutionize the field. In this chapter, we will provide a concise summary of the key findings in materials science and engineering related to tissue engineering, offering insights into the advancements that are propelling us towards a better tomorrow.

One of the most significant findings in this field is the development of biomaterials that can mimic the natural extracellular matrix (ECM) of tissues. The ECM is a complex network of proteins and other molecules that provide structural support and regulate cell behavior. Researchers have successfully engineered biomaterials that replicate the ECM's composition, allowing for improved cell adhesion, proliferation, and differentiation. This breakthrough has paved the way for the creation of artificial tissues and organs that closely resemble their natural counterparts.

Another important finding is the discovery of innovative scaffold designs. Scaffolds are three-dimensional structures that provide a framework for cells to grow and organize. Researchers have explored various scaffold architectures, such as porous structures, fibers, and hydrogels, to optimize cell attachment, nutrient diffusion, and waste removal. These advancements have led to the development of scaffolds that can support tissue regeneration in complex organs, such as the heart and liver.

In addition to biomaterials and scaffolds, the field of tissue engineering has witnessed significant progress in the realm of cell sources. Stem cells, particularly induced pluripotent stem cells (iPSCs), have emerged as a promising cell source due to their ability to differentiate into various cell types. Researchers have successfully directed the differentiation of iPSCs into specific cell lineages, offering a renewable and patient-specific cell source for tissue engineering applications.

Furthermore, innovative manufacturing techniques have played a pivotal role in advancing tissue engineering. Additive manufacturing, commonly known as 3D printing, has revolutionized the fabrication of complex tissue constructs with precise control over architecture and composition. This technology allows researchers to create patient-specific implants and organs, reducing the risk of rejection and improving overall treatment outcomes.

Overall, the key findings summarized in this chapter highlight the remarkable progress made in materials science and engineering for tissue engineering applications. These discoveries bring us closer to a future where damaged tissues and organs can be regenerated or replaced, offering hope for patients suffering from various medical conditions. By combining the expertise from materials science and engineering with the principles of tissue engineering, we are building a better tomorrow for everyone.

Promising Developments and Emerging Trends

In the fast-paced world of materials science and engineering, innovations are constantly reshaping the landscape of tissue engineering. The field of tissue engineering aims to create functional, viable tissues and organs to replace or repair damaged ones. This subchapter explores the promising developments and emerging trends that are revolutionizing the future of tissue engineering and building a better tomorrow for patients worldwide.

One of the most exciting developments in tissue engineering is the advent of 3D bioprinting. This groundbreaking technology allows researchers to precisely deposit cells, biomaterials, and growth factors layer by layer, creating intricate structures that mimic the complexity of natural tissues. With the ability to print organs and tissues on-demand, 3D bioprinting holds immense potential to address the growing demand for organ transplantation and eliminate the need for donor waiting lists.

Another area showing promise is the use of stem cells in tissue engineering. Stem cells possess the remarkable ability to differentiate into various cell types, making them ideal for constructing complex tissues. Recent advancements in stem cell research have led to the development of induced pluripotent stem cells (iPSCs), which can be derived from adult cells and reprogrammed into a pluripotent state. iPSCs offer an ethical and patient-specific approach to tissue engineering, bypassing the need for donor tissues and reducing the risk of rejection.

Nanotechnology is also playing a vital role in tissue engineering. By manipulating materials at the nanoscale, scientists can create scaffolds with enhanced mechanical properties, tailored surface topographies, and controlled drug delivery systems. Nanomaterials, such as graphene and carbon nanotubes, have shown great potential in promoting cell adhesion, proliferation, and differentiation. Furthermore, nanotechnology enables the development of smart materials that respond to external stimuli like pH, temperature, or electrical signals, facilitating tissue regeneration and repair.

Additionally, advancements in biomaterials have opened new horizons in tissue engineering. Scaffold materials with improved biocompatibility, mechanical strength, and degradation profiles are being developed to provide optimal support for cell growth and tissue formation. Biomimetic materials, inspired by the native extracellular matrix, are being designed to recreate the biochemical and mechanical cues necessary for proper tissue development. These innovative biomaterials hold great promise in regenerating damaged tissues and promoting functional integration with the host.

In conclusion, the field of tissue engineering is witnessing promising developments and emerging trends that hold tremendous potential for building a better tomorrow. From 3D bioprinting and stem cell research to nanotechnology and advanced biomaterials, researchers are revolutionizing the way we approach tissue regeneration and organ replacement. By harnessing these advancements, we can envision a future where personalized, functional tissues and organs are readily available, revolutionizing the healthcare industry and improving the quality of life for countless individuals.

Impact of Tissue Engineering on Healthcare

Tissue engineering has emerged as a revolutionary field that combines materials science and engineering principles to develop innovative solutions for enhancing healthcare outcomes. By harnessing the power of biomaterials, cells, and biophysical factors, tissue engineering aims to regenerate or repair damaged tissues and organs, ultimately providing hope for patients worldwide. This subchapter delves into the profound impact that tissue engineering has had on healthcare, with a specific focus on the materials science and engineering aspects driving its success.

One of the key contributions of tissue engineering is the development of biocompatible materials that can mimic the natural extracellular matrix (ECM) found in tissues. These materials provide a supportive environment for cells to adhere, proliferate, and differentiate, facilitating tissue regeneration. Researchers have engineered a wide range of biomaterials, including polymers, hydrogels, ceramics, and composites, each with unique properties tailored to specific tissue requirements. For instance, biodegradable scaffolds made from polymers can provide mechanical support during tissue regeneration, gradually degrading as the new tissue forms.

Moreover, tissue engineering has opened up new possibilities in the field of regenerative medicine. It has enabled the creation of artificial organs and tissues, reducing the burden on organ transplantation waiting lists. Complex organs like the heart, kidney, and liver can be developed using a combination of biomaterials, cells, and bioreactors. These bioengineered organs have the potential to overcome the limitations of donor scarcity and immune rejection, offering a promising solution for patients in need.

In addition to organ replacement, tissue engineering has also revolutionized the field of drug testing and personalized medicine. Traditional drug testing methods using animal models often fail to accurately predict human responses. Tissue-engineered models, such as organ-on-a-chip systems, allow researchers to study the effects of drugs on human tissues more accurately. This enables the development of safer and more effective drugs, tailored to individual patients, thereby reducing the risk of adverse reactions.

The impact of tissue engineering on healthcare extends beyond regenerative medicine and drug testing. It has also played a vital role in the advancement of wound healing, including chronic wounds and burns. By developing smart dressings and scaffolds that release growth factors and promote cell migration, tissue engineering has significantly improved wound healing outcomes, reducing the risk of infection and scarring.

In conclusion, tissue engineering has revolutionized healthcare by merging materials science and engineering principles with biology. The field has made significant strides in regenerative medicine, organ transplantation, drug testing, and wound healing. The continuous advancements in biomaterials and tissue engineering techniques hold immense potential for building a better tomorrow in healthcare, providing hope for patients and improving their quality of life.

The Role of Materials in Shaping a Better Tomorrow

Introduction:
In the quest for a better tomorrow, materials science and engineering play a crucial role. From revolutionizing the way we live to addressing pressing global challenges, the right materials have the power to shape a brighter future. This subchapter explores the pivotal role of materials in various aspects of society, ranging from healthcare to energy and sustainability.

Materials in Healthcare:
Medical advancements heavily rely on the development of innovative materials. From biocompatible implants to tissue engineering scaffolds, materials science has revolutionized the field of healthcare. These materials enable the repair and regeneration of damaged tissues and organs, providing hope to millions of patients worldwide. With ongoing research, the possibilities for improved medical treatments and personalized healthcare are expanding rapidly.

Materials in Energy:
The search for clean and sustainable energy sources is another critical area where materials science plays a significant role. Advanced materials have paved the way for the development of more efficient solar cells, lightweight batteries, and fuel cells. These innovations offer a path towards reducing our dependence on fossil fuels and mitigating the impact of climate change. The ongoing research in materials science holds immense potential for creating a greener and more sustainable energy future.

Materials in Environmental Sustainability: The materials we use daily can have a significant impact on the environment. Sustainable materials, such as biodegradable polymers and recyclable composites, are key to reducing waste and minimizing our carbon footprint. By designing materials with a focus on eco-friendliness and durability, we can contribute to a more sustainable future. Furthermore, materials science is exploring ways to develop materials that can actively remove pollutants from the air and water, offering potential solutions to pressing environmental challenges.

Conclusion:

Materials science and engineering have an undeniable impact on shaping a better tomorrow. From healthcare to energy and environmental sustainability, the right materials can revolutionize industries and improve the quality of life for people worldwide. As we continue to push the boundaries of materials research, it is essential to collaborate across disciplines and invest in innovative solutions. By harnessing the potential of materials, we can build a future that is characterized by progress, sustainability, and improved well-being for all.

www.ingramcontent.com/pod-product-compliance
Lightning Source LLC
LaVergne TN
LVHW010225070526
838199LV00062B/4727